£1.75

A Village in Chelsea
An informal account of the Royal Hospital

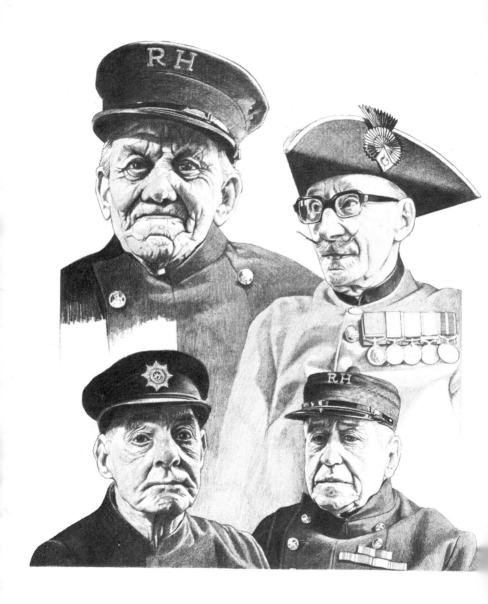

FOUR FACES OF CHELSEA

A Village
in Chelsea

An informal account of the Royal Hospital

by David Ascoli

With illustrations by
Andrew Farmer

WILLIAM LUSCOMBE PUBLISHER LIMITED
(in association with Mitchell Beazley Limited)

First published in Great Britain
by William Luscombe Publisher Ltd
The Mitchell Beazley Group
Artists House
14–15 Manette Street,
London W1V 5LB
1974

ISBN 0 86002 037 1

Printed Offset Litho in Great Britain by
Cox & Wyman Ltd,
London, Fakenham and Reading

*Dedicated with pride and affection
to the old gentlemen themselves,
the In-Pensioners of the Royal Hospital*

Contents

Illustrations

IN SUBSIDIUM ET LEVAMEN
EMERITORUM SENIO BELLOQUE
FRACTORUM CONDIDIT
CAROLUS SECUNDUS,
AUXIT JACOBUS SECUNDUS,
PERFECERE GULIELMUS ET MARIA,
REX ET REGINA – MDCXCII

A note on comparative money values

In this account of the Royal Hospital there will be numerous references to salary and pension levels and to the cost of such items as food and clothing over the past three hundred years. These figures are meaningless to the average reader unless they can be related to the present-day pound sterling. Exact comparisons are impossible since for the years before the First World War statistics are very imprecise and based on a very small selection of commodities. Furthermore, the figures are distorted by the incidence of income tax and excise duty. For example, a hundred years ago a bottle of whisky cost 3s. and a reasonable claret 1s. 6d. It was possible for a family of six to have a very cheerful Christmas dinner indeed for an outlay of under 16s. on drink.* An identical 'sideboard' would cost £16·70 today! Nonetheless it is possible to arrive at a broadly accurate comparison; and here it is. I have shown the value of the 1974 £ at various key dates in the history of the Royal Hospital:

1681	£14·50
1692	£15·20
1715	£13·30
1783	£11·10
1815	£5·70
1833	£7·70
1847	£8·10
1870	£7·10
1894	£8·90
1920	£3·40

* 1	× Whisky	3s.
1	× Brandy	3s.
1	× Sherry	1s. 2d.
1	× Port	1s. 3d.
3	× Claret	4s. 6d.
2	× Sauternes	2s. 10d.
		15s. 9d.

1930	£5·10
1946	£3·20
1960	£2·10

This table tells its own story: a progressive erosion of the pound during the eighteenth century culminating in massive inflation during the Napoleonic wars; a period of remarkable stability during Victoria's reign until the largely forgotten depression of the 1890s; after 1918 another savage period of inflation until the Great Depression of the 1930s; after the Second World War a return to inflation which, like the poor, seems now to be always with us. While the pound went through its ritual dances, no one seems to have remembered the Royal Hospital. For over 250 years the Governor's salary was pegged at £500 a year and In-Pensioners' subsistence at 8*d.* a week,* while for 120 years the basic rate of out-pension remained unchanged at 5*d.* a day. And, as we shall see, these were by no means the only curiosities.

* From 1902 to 1931 the figure was actually *reduced* to 7*d.*

Introduction

It is twenty-five years since Capt. Dean's history of the Royal Hospital was published. Graham Dean spent thirty-four years of his life at Chelsea, twenty-one of them as a Captain of Invalids and thirteen as Adjutant. He loved the place and became a considerable authority on Sir Christopher Wren and on the social and political background of the Hospital. His book is the *locus classicus* for all students of the subject.

Dean's approach, however, was quite different from my own. His book, the product of detailed and meticulous research, is a somewhat dry and formal history and was not intended to cover the human aspect of the Hospital, which is one of the liveliest and most colourful of our national institutions. This is a pity, for the archives are anything but dry and formal – and the In-Pensioners even less so! Year by year, down the centuries, these archives record the humour and melancholy of life in all its odd diversity. Here, for example, is the still unknown Edgar Wallace writing from the *Evening News* staff office in 1905 to suggest a visit of ten In-Pensioner veterans of the Crimean War to meet their opposite numbers in the Invalides in Paris, 'with all expenses defrayed as befits our heroes of far-off campaigns'. The Commissioners thought otherwise: 'It was unanimously agreed that this highly undesirable invitation should be rejected out of hand.' Times have changed. Today the In-Pensioners travel away not only to the Invalides and the Soldiers' Home in Washington, but to Laurel Park racetrack, to their regiments at home and abroad, and to sons and daughters in Canada and far-off Australia.

As a privileged outsider, it has seemed to me that the In-Pensioners of Chelsea are more important than the stage on which they have acted out their dramas and their comedies. And so I have given them pride of place. It has been a highly diverting experience. I have learned a great deal about the Royal Hospital. But I have learned a great deal more about the nature and quality of old soldiers. And so primarily this is a book about people, both great and humble. And since it takes all sorts to make a world, it is a book about both saints and sinners. The Royal Hospital would be a dull place without the one; it would be a great deal duller without the other!

While writing this book I have found myself constantly wishing that tape-recorders had existed at the time of Blenheim or Dettingen or Waterloo to capture the thoughts and experiences of those blunt but illiterate veterans. So I have tried to make amends by recording the lives and adventures of some twenty-five old soldiers of the present day so that the tapes may be preserved in the Hospital museum. I chose In-Pensioners from different regiments and from widely separated parts of the country (unintentionally the result is an audio-library of the regional accents of the British Isles!). Unlike their distant predecessors, the old gentlemen to-day are both literate and articulate, and blessed with remarkable memories.

For example: Bert Turp, Farrier-Sergeant of the Royals, born in 1885 in a pub in South Ockendon ('my mother was there at the time'), who enlisted on St Patrick's Day *seventy-two years ago*; 'Micky' Rooney, aged 84, of the Border Regiment, who gave up a job in the Whitehaven pits 'because Sunday shift work interfered with my courting'; George Batty of the 17/21st Lancers, who as a boy *walked* from Salford to Blackpool to sell newspapers and run errands and lost every penny he earned playing brag, and who forty years later was a valet at the Savoy; Charlie Mitchell of the RHA, from Battersea, who had a nanny to look after him until 'my father had some differences with racehorses and went broke', and whose subsequent army rank, in his own words, 'went up and down like a yo-yo'; 'Jockey' Frere, D.C.M., of the 3rd Hussars, who died a month short of his 91st birthday and left £11,000 to the Royal Hospital.

Always funny, often touching, the stories of these old soldiers and others like them deserve a book to themselves. We shall meet some of them in due course.

I am greatly indebted to many people. First and foremost, to the present Governor, General Sir Charles Jones, who has given me unique facilities and the freedom of the Royal Hospital, and who has encouraged and helped me in every way. I owe him a greater debt than perhaps he knows and I hope this book may justify all his kindness and consideration.

There are many others. General Sir Frank Simpson, the previous Governor, one of the great servants of the Royal Hospital and a mine of information and anecdote. John Le Mesurier, who was Adjutant when I first came upon the scene, and who opened all sorts of improbable doors for me. To him and Joanna I owe a special debt. The legendary Jimmie Ives, who was R.S.M. at Chelsea for nineteen years and who knows more about the In-Pensioners than either he – or they – would care to admit! And the whole staff of the Hospital, from Major-General Morrison, Physician and Surgeon, to the cheerful *senoritas* of the Great Hall who have attended so kindly to my creature comforts day by day – three courses, 18p a time.

But above all, I am indebted to the old gentlemen themselves. They have filled my house and garden with colour and great good humour. They have filled me with good whisky and tall stories in their Club. And they have filled me at all times with a great sense of pride in the old and stable virtues of dignity, courtesy and discipline.

My researches have taken me not only to the Royal Hospital, but also to the Hôtel des Invalides in Paris, the Public Record Office, Chelsea Public Library, the National Army Museum, the Imperial War Museum, and to many other more remote corners. In particular, I recall a pleasant hour with the Duke of St Albans, discussing his celebrated forebear, Nell Gwyn. For the rest, I have preferred to let the Royal Hospital speak for itself. After all, even old soldiers have been known to blush.

D.N.A.

Pilgrim's Cottage,
Shalford,
1974.

I

'So exelent a worke...'

In subsidium et levamen emeritorum
senio belloque fractorum.

Of all London's historic institutions, the Royal Hospital is one of the least known and least frequented by visitors; and this is curious. Despite the passage of time and the ravages of war, the main fabric of Wren's grand design is largely unaltered from that Spring day in 1692 when the first In-Pensioners took up residence; and it still honours faithfully the purpose of its 'pious founder', Charles II. Unlike most national monuments, it is no museum of antique buildings, but a living and a lived-in place; and in this it shares an unique distinction with our ancient seats of learning. Yet whereas they were devoted to the advancement of the young, the Royal Hospital was, and is, dedicated to the help and comfort of the old.

There is no existing record of all those old soldiers – *'emeritorum senio belloque fractorum'* – who have lived and died in the Long Wards at Chelsea, but we can do some arithmetic. The original establishment laid down in 1682 by Stephen Fox, the first 'director-general' of the Hospital and arguably its greatest benefactor, was for '422 military persons'. This figure has fluctuated in proportion to the nation's involvement in war, and to the parsimony – or peculation – of those set in authority. If, however, we take an average complement of 450, and if we accept an actuarial average of seven years from entry to death, then the total roll-call is of the order of 18,000. They are therefore a very exclusive élite.

The comparative 'remoteness' of the Royal Hospital may possibly arise from its name, and from the popular belief that it is a strictly medical institution and thus, as it were, an enclosed order. Nothing could be further from the truth. The word 'hospital' was used by Charles in his original Royal Warrant in its old and proper sense of 'a place of refuge and shelter' and, as we shall see, the foundation was simply a development, on an entirely novel scale, of the mediaeval almshouse. It is, in effect, a self-contained village centred around its own chapel, its communal dining-hall, its infirmary, its post office, and its social club – a community of old gentlemen with

17

similar backgrounds and like experiences. And like any self-respecting village, it thrives on the gossip of the parish-pump. Nowhere does news travel faster. Nowhere does fact acquire a more intricate embroidery of fiction. It is indeed the last repository of old soldiers' tales.

The story of the Royal Hospital is, in a sense, a microcosm of our social scene across three centuries; and despite many vicissitudes, it has survived the several shocks of gross mismanagement and political animosity. Above all, it remains a lasting memorial to its great author. There can be few places more perfectly tempered to 'that unhoped serene that men call age'. Charles Burney, who was organist in the Chapel from 1783 to 1814, described it as a quiet retreat where 'none goes at above a foot-pace'; and the early files of the Adjutant's Journal repeatedly invoke the spirit of tranquillity: 'Whatever Centinel neglects these Orders will be punished, as will also that at the Cupola who shall suffer Boys to run about, spoil the Walks and throw Stones at the Statue.'

Until as recently as 1955 the Royal Hospital was responsible for the administration of all Army pensions, and for a century and a half, Out-Pensioners were required to attend in person at Chelsea twice a year to draw their money (if they were lucky) and to be re-examined for continued admission to the out-pension list. On first admission, men had to wait twelve months before drawing the money due to them and thereafter, at least technically, pensions were paid half-yearly in arrears, a system that led to gross abuses.

The tone was set by Richard Jones, first Earl of Ranelagh, Paymaster-General from 1685 to 1702, and one of the prize villains of an age when villainy was an accomplished art. His method was classically simple and consisted of embezzling such sums as were made available for the payment of Out-Pensioners, while at the same time virtually closing the list to new admissions until by 1702 the number had fallen to the derisory figure of fifty-one. After seventeen years of largely undetected crime, he was finally rumbled, dismissed from his lucrative post and expelled from the House of Commons. There is little doubt that he was the evil genius of the Hospital's early years and we shall examine his shady record more fully in due course.

The abuse of the pension fund reached even greater excesses during Robert Walpole's administration, for by then all and sundry, from recruiting-sergeants to the Secretary and the Deputy Treasurer of the Hospital, had got in on the act. Not only were old soldiers charged illicit fees for admission to the pension list (since Marlborough's wars, the numbers had increased dramatically), but a flourishing business in moneylending grew up by which Out-Pensioners could obtain an advance at interest rates varying between 8 per cent and 34 per cent. In 1715 the position had become so serious that a Committee of Inquiry of the Privy Council reported '. . . that there are recruiting officers that bear up for and levy invalids to claim the pension: there are officers that prepare the certificates of the men's qualifications, Furlows signed by the governor are always ready for them immediately upon their admission to the pension list, and there are persons ready to take upon them the trouble of receiving their pension by letter of attorney, and to advance to them as the stock rises and falls in and about Chelsea.' The In-Pensioners had the last laugh for they at least had surrendered their pension rights against free board and lodging and a modest subsistence allowance.

Predictably nothing came of the Inquiry and the irregularities persisted even after Walpole's resignation and the arrival of William Pitt at the Pay Office in 1746. Indeed, it took that honest man eight years to hit upon the simple solution of paying out-pensions half-yearly in advance.

The fact that all pensions were administered from Chelsea is reflected in the Hospital archives which, instead of recording purely parochial affairs, open a succession of windows on the world outside. Here are some random vignettes, each a tiny facet of the humour, the melancholy, and the absurdity of life.

On March 12, 1774, Samuel Quinn, a 'greatly lacerated' soldier of the 12th Foot, was 'dismist the Royal Hospital in that he did wantonly set fire to his uniform'. This is arguably one of the first recorded instances of that time-honoured cry: 'I'll soldier no more!'

In 1806, the clerks in the Secretary's office submitted a petition for a salary increase (such requests occur with monotonous regularity in the Chelsea Board Minutes). But there is a familiar ring about their peroration: 'They therefore humbly hope that your Lordships will be pleased to take their cases into consideration, particularly the great difference in every Article of life, compared with the Price a few Years back.' And there is an even more familiar ring about the Board's decision: 'Refer to next meeting.'

On May 14, 1848, Thomas Morgan, late of the 14th Dragoons, Out-Pensioner at 1*s.* a day, submitted a request for an increase in his pension, supported by a medical certificate which stated that he suffered from 'dyspnoea, rupture, rheumatism, varicose veins and incontinence of urine'. The Board's decision was curt and dismissive: 'Insufficient cause.'

The Chelsea Board, when occasion demanded, could demonstrate their gallantry under fire. After the death of the Duke of Wellington in 1852, a communication was received from the Queen 'enquiring' (a Royal euphemism, this) whether his 'funeral car' might be put on permanent public display in the Great Hall. After due deliberation the Board replied that in their opinion 'this proposal would be a source of serious inconvenience to the In-Pensioners, whose interest must be considered paramount'; and duly declined Her Majesty's most gracious suggestion. Brave words, indeed!

On November 12, 1857, the Board was notified that Henry Johnson, Out-Pensioner, late of the 55th Foot, had been convicted in the Chatham Court of the theft of 'a hank of horsehair'. The Board duly minuted: 'To be struck off the Pension List.' And for this insignificant crime, the unfortunate Johnson was sentenced to 'transportation for life'.

In November, 1858, the Board was informed that Thomas Solly, aged 82, late of the Horse Artillery, In-Pensioner at 1*s*. a day, 'is most anxious to revert to Out-Pension as his daughter is married to a Missionary at the Cape, wishes him to join them there and the emigrant ship in which he proposes going will sail shortly.' To which the Board replied: 'Agreed. Pension to be paid in future at the Cape of Good Hope.' One wonders how old Tom Solly fared.

In January, 1893, the Physician and Surgeon was authorized to procure the following 'usual quarterly supply of Wines and Spirits for Sick Pensioners in the Infirmary':

9 dozen	Port Wine
10 dozen	Gin
10 dozen	Brandy
10 dozen	Whisky
2 dozen	Soda Water (Schweppes)

Eleven days later a note in the Minutes records that there was a 'substantial waiting-list for admission to the Infirmary'. One can see why.

On October 10, 1945, the Board approved an increase in the existing grant for the choir from £150 to £210 a year 'to improve (its) volume and quality', subject to review after one year. Not only the 'volume and quality' improved. By 1972 the choir was costing £1,000 a year.

It is impossible to turn the pages of these years, each recorded in an elegant and faultless copper-plate hand, without being greatly moved by distant echoes of the human comedy. What manner of men were these who sought a modest reputation in the cannon's mouth and then came at the end to live out their autumn days in the peace and quiet of Chelsea? For the most part they were unknown soldiers, for few could read and fewer still could write. But between them, saints and sinners alike, they helped to build an Empire and we know enough about them to be sure that they were men of character and courage. We shall meet them as we go, and we shall recognize in them the same warm blood and good humour that walks the Colonnade today.

When, in 1682, Wren embarked upon the building of the Hospital on the site of the abandoned Chelsea College, Chelsea itself was a village of some 300 inhabitants, set in open country, a fifteen minute coach ride from Westminster. In course of time the Commissioners acquired much of the surrounding land so that today the Hospital is an island of repose whose shores are washed by an urban sea.

There have been critics of Wren's architectural achievement at Chelsea. That is a matter of personal taste. Wotan no doubt had his critics when Valhalla was built, and the Royal Hospital has much in common with Valhalla. But to savour its monumental quality, the visitor must stand at the northern end of Burton's Court and let his fantasy range across three hundred years when all around was green and the grand enclosure swept down through Figure Court, through ornamental gardens, to the riverside. This noble design owed much to the royal palaces of France where Wren first learned the rudiments of his craft.

The building of the Hospital took ten years, and extended over three reigns. It was embellished in the eighteenth century by Robert Adam, and disfigured in the nineteenth by John Soane. Thereafter it remained virtually untouched until in two World Wars it suffered grievous damage by enemy action. Today the scars of war have healed and a splendid new Infirmary stands where General Wilford's estate once thwarted previous developers. Gone are the elegant residences which Ranelagh and Sir Robert Walpole built for themselves out of misappropriated public funds. Gone is the Rotunda, William Jones's stately pleasure-dome in Ranelagh Gardens. Greenwich and Kilmainham have long since closed their doors to pensioners, the one for disciplinary, the other for political reasons. Chelsea alone remains.

Yet in time the changing image of the Hospital and of its In-Pensioners has reflected the shifts in the prevailing winds of the day, whether political, military or social. The eighteenth century was the age of the 'brutal and licentious soldiery', and contemporary artists, almost without exception, represented the pensioners as Hogarthian figures or characters from the *Beggars' Opera*. This was not as uncharitable as it may seem. A high proportion of men admitted at that time were crippled by wounds or other infirmities, and few survived to qualify solely by virtue of old age.

One such was the celebrated William Hiseland who died in 1732 at the age of 112 and today lies in the Burial Ground. This splendid character served the Crown for upwards of eighty years, from Edgehill to Blenheim and beyond, and entered the Royal Hospital in 1713. Even then there was life in the old dog yet for, as the inscription on his tomb tells us, 'What rendered his Age still more Patriarchal, when above one Hundred Years old He took unto Him a wife'. Indeed, if we may judge from contemporary records, the veterans of that day may have lost their limbs, but certainly not their virility.*

The eighteenth century was also the high point of the Royal Hospital as a centre of social life. The festival dinners at the Governor's Table were notable occasions and attracted, among many others, James Boswell and his circle, while the neighbouring Ranelagh Gardens (they were not re-acquired by the Chelsea Board until 1826) became the favourite place of entertainment for London society and, in the end, notorious for 'carousals of the most depraved kind'. What the old soldiers thought of all this is not recorded, but since the breed does not change, we may readily surmise.

---

* Longevity seems to have been a feature of the Royal Hospital, as the following list of eighteenth-century veterans shows:

	Died	Age
Thomas Azbey	1737	112
'Captain' Laurence	1765	95
Robert Cumming	1767	116
Peter Dowling	1768	102
'A soldier who		
fought at the		
battle of the Boyne'	1772	111
Peter Bennet	1773	107

By the nineteenth century the image had changed again. The Napoleonic wars and the succession of Imperial campaigns which followed resulted in a considerable increase in applications for admission to the Hospital. But in Victorian England a scarlet coat was unremarkable, and by the middle of the century the In-Pensioners suffered the same public disesteem in which the Army had come to be held. It is indicative that between 1870 and 1894 three abortive inquiries were held to examine the possibility – and desirability – of closing the Hospital down.

The previous century had been the Age of Cynicism. The Victorian era was the Age of Sentiment. And so contemporary artists, almost without exception, represented the In-Pensioners as bearded patricians, often in the company of small and wondering children. And this, too, was not as uncharitable as it may seem.

Our own century has seen a much more radical change. After the First World War, nothing could ever be the same again, and this was particularly true of the Royal Hospital; for this was the Age of Disillusion, and ex-servicemen have always been among the first victims of a mood of national disenchantment. It is probably true to say that in the years between the wars, the Hospital touched the lowest point in its fortunes. Old soldiers came to look upon the place as a glorified poor-house. The public came to look upon the In-Pensioners as 'beggars in scarlet'. Both were wrong, yet little was done at Chelsea to put the record straight.

But in Montaigne's phrase 'great institutions survive little men , and the post-war years have seen the Royal Hospital recover its proud and ancient standing. The British are a curious people, most unpredictable when every prediction seems clear. Possibly the Hospital is the beneficiary of a national feeling of nostalgia at the retreat from Empire. Certainly it is the beneficiary of a succession of dedicated Governors. But there are other more subtle reasons which we shall examine in due course.

No institution, however august or revered, can long endure in the face of public disapproval, and today the public has a warm affection for its Chelsea Pensioners. Yet the public knows remarkably little about them – who they are, how they come to be there, how they live, their origins and their traditions. Certainly there are those to whom the Royal Hospital is an anachronism in a modern world. If that is so, then all tradition – Church, Crown, even the State itself – is anachronism. In recent years envious eyes have been cast at Wren's great building and its suitability for other, less worthy purposes. It has survived for three centuries to provide 'help and comfort for old soldiers broken by age and war'. It will not, one suspects, surrender easily.

In an age that mocks the virtues of service and discipline, it is well to be reminded of these enduring qualities. This book, then, is a tribute to the honourable profession of arms, to the honourable upholders of that tradition, and to the British genius for survival. And last but not least, it is a tribute to the memory of a King who, though he may never have said a foolish thing, certainly did one wise one.

2

'We have a pretty witty King . . .'

On May 29, 1660, his thirtieth birthday, Charles II re-entered London in triumph. John Evelyn watched the royal progress from the Strand: 'This day, his Majesty, Charles the Second came to London, after a sad and long exile and calamitous suffering, being seventeen years . . . with a triumph of above 20,000 horse and foot, brandishing their swords and shouting with inexpressible joy; the ways strewed with flowers, the bells ringing, the streets hung with tapestry, fountains running with wine . . . trumpets, music, and myriads of people flocking, even so far as from Rochester, so as they were seven hours in passing the city, even from two in the afternoon till nine at night . . . And all this was done without one drop of blood shed, and by that very army which rebelled against him.'

And to match the occasion, the sun shone with regal splendour. It had been a long, dark night.

The England to which Charles returned was wearied by years of civil war and drained of spirit by the effects of a grey Puritanism totally alien to the rough, good-humoured English character. The eleven years between the execution of Charles I and the restoration of his son are unique in our history. The Civil War had arisen from a head-on collision between two inflexible principles: that of a King convinced that his divine right and his royal prerogatives – in short, the principle of absolute monarchy – should prevail; and that of a Parliament determined that all power proceeded from the people who were the masters and not the servants of Church and State.

The vacuum left by the abolition of the monarchy was filled – or, more exactly, occupied – by Oliver Cromwell, a man often as indecisive in affairs of state as he had been decisive in battle, a prisoner at once of his own Englishness and of the military weapon he had helped to forge. He stands before us in history as a flawed man, believing in the sanctity of property yet ready to condone its appropriation; preaching 'liberty of conscience' yet permitting the persecution of both Roman and Anglican church alike; a republican at heart, yet a monarch in all but name.

Nonetheless he remains a great Englishman who, though he

presided over a military dictatorship, held fast to his concept of freedom and rebuilt the prestige and standing of his country as much by his own example as by his achievements in foreign policy. No other man of his time could have contained the passions of the day, or kept a factious parliament and an arrogant army from each other's throats; and at his death in 1658, there were only two options open to the country – a return to bloodshed or a return to monarchy. The country opted for restoration, but the echoes of the Interregnum were to resound not only down the years of Charles II's reign, but to the present day. And not least this is true of the growth and development of the Regular Army.

Life during the Republic was without colour and devoid of humour, to the astonishment of the French ambassador who reported: 'I did not think a lively people could be so shortly sunk in apathy.' National sports and pastimes such as horse-racing and maypole-dancing were banned, the one for fear of public disorder, the other for fear of immorality. Theatres were closed and throughout the Interregnum no single play of Shakespeare was publicly performed. And while one voice was stilled, another – that of John Milton – thundered through the land, summoning people to the contemplation of the wages of sin. The property of Crown, Church and royalist landowners was sequestrated or sold at nominal cost to Parliamentary grandees, and church buildings were desecrated with a fine disregard for Puritan professions of godliness; a renegade knight of the shires removed the stained-glass windows of Westminster Abbey and Cromwell's troopers stabled their horses in St Paul's.

Adultery was a crime punishable by death (the mind boggles at the rivers of blood which would have flowed in Charles's permissive society, had this law not been suspended). Drunkenness was prosecuted with zeal, and ale-houses, the most English of institutions, were circumscribed and severely rationed. 'To drink,' wrote a contemporary, 'is become a most sober occupation.' Swearing was punished by a neatly graduated scale of fines: a duke paid 30s. for a first offence, a baron 20s. and a squire 10s. Common people could relieve their feelings for 3s. 4d., which represented ten days' average wages. To which Winston Churchill has added a wry comment: 'Not much was allowed for their money; one man was fined for saying "God is my witness", and another for saying "Upon my life".'

All forms of extravagance in dress were frowned upon and laws were passed forbidding the wearing of any jewellery or ornaments.

The festivals of the church calendar were singled out as special targets by the self-appointed keepers of public morals and the muted celebration of Christmas was conducted under the baleful eye of vice-squads of the soldiery. Beside all this, the Puritanism of Victorian England seems like an exercise in cheerful debauchery.

After so long a winter of discontent, it is not surprising that the return of a young, attractive King should have been the occasion for national rejoicing such as Evelyn witnessed. Even during the darkest days of the Protectorate, the royalist fires had burned steadily, for the idea of kingship and of rule by law established had survived centuries of discord and the people, having experienced the odour of Puritan sanctity and the iron fist of Cromwell's major-generals, were passionately determined that 'the King should enjoy his own again'. In the twenty-five years that followed the Restoration, the country twice came again to the brink of civil war. But the nation – King, peers and commoners – had once looked into the abyss; and faced again with the same grim prospect, and with the benefit of hindsight that the earlier generation had not known, they stepped back from the edge.

The festival spirit that attended the King's return was short-lived. In 1661 Charles summoned his new Parliament. It was to last for eighteen stormy years, the longest life of any Parliament in our history. It is remembered as the Cavalier Parliament, but it had another, less attractive face – that of the Pension Parliament. For by the end of its life, at least half its members were in the pay of Louis XIV and most of the remainder were in receipt of Dutch bribes.

Charles's reign falls into a distinct pattern, coloured throughout by the refusal of Parliament to grant him an adequate supply of money with which to conduct the affairs of state. When the Commons met in 1661, they voted him the sum of £1,200,000 a year based on a totally inaccurate estimate of the yield from customs and excise, supplemented by various financial expedients such as a duty on wines, the unpopular hearth tax and minor irrelevancies like the hackney carriage licence revenue. Throughout his reign, income fell far short of expenditure, despite various supplementary votes to finance the conduct of the two Dutch Wars. And at no time was any provision made for settlement of the massive debts which he inherited. It is greatly to his credit that, however strait his circumstances, the King considered the reduction of those debts as his chief priority, even when the standing revenue of the Crown was severely reduced by the disasters of the Great Plague and the Fire of London. It is all the more remarkable that towards the end of his life, when he had decided to rule without a Parliament and therefore without a constitutional source of revenue, he still went forward with the grand and costly project for his Hospital at Chelsea. How ingeniously this was financed during a period of widespread public retrenchment is a subject to which we will return.

The refusal of Parliament to provide Charles with an adequate revenue had far-reaching consequences. The first of these was to engender a growing bitterness between King and Commons which culminated in the final dissolution of 1681. Secondly it drove the King into a devious and ultimately dangerous association with the Catholic King of France. Charles's critics have made much of the proposition that he sold his country's foreign policy for a mess of French pottage. This is partly true, for by nature and upbringing Charles was strongly pro-French, and admired – and envied – his French cousin. But of the £1,000,000 that Charles received from Louis by way of subsidy, or bribe, or hush-money, by far the greater proportion was spent on strengthening the Royal Navy and thus creating an instrument not only for the defence of the realm but for the expansion and security of the colonial empire on which the power and influence of England was shortly to rest. During his reign, Charles met and addressed his 'faithful' Commons forty-eight times. On virtually every occasion, he asked them to vote him an additional supply for the building of more ships and for the betterment of the Fleet. For example, on November 20, 1661:

'I come to put you in mind . . . of the great sum of money that should be ready to discharge the several Fleets when they come home; and for the necessary preparations that are to be made for the setting out new fleets to sea against the spring.'

And seventeen years later there is an unusual note of exasperation:

'So I must tell you . . . that if you would have me pass any part of my life in ease or quiet, and all the rest of it in perfect confidence and kindness with you and all succeeding Parliaments; you must find a way of settling for my life, not only my revenue, and the additional duties as they were at Christmas last, but of adding to them, upon some new funds, £300,000 a year. Upon which I shall consent that an Act may pass for appropriating

£500,000 a year to the constant maintenance of the Navy and Ordnance, which I take to be the greatest safety and interest of these kingdoms.'

Not once in all these years did Charles specifically ask for an additional supply to maintain that standing army which Parliament held in such hatred and suspicion, except, ironically, on March 6, 1679 when, under pressure from the opposition, he informed them that

'I have disbanded as much of the Army *as I could get money to do*; and I am ready to disband the rest, so soon as you shall reimburse what they have cost me, and will enable me to pay off the remainder.'

Predictably, Parliament did not reimburse him.

This particular passage of arms had one significant result. The disbanding of a large part of the army raised a major matter of principle. The arrangements for resettling superannuated or redundant soldiers into civilian life at that time were purely haphazard; and while the refusal of Parliament to match the King's reasonable offer meant that the run-down of the army was left to Charles's discretion, nonetheless some four thousand soldiers found themselves without occupation or pension rights. As such, they were a potential danger to public order and an undesirable charge upon parish funds, and so it can fairly be said that the intransigence of the Commons in 1679 created the situation out of which, two years later, the Royal Hospital was born.

But money was not the only bone of contention between King and Parliament. Far more explosive – because it was a national rather than a personal issue – was the religious confrontation.

In the Declaration of Breda which Charles drew up under the direction of the future Earl of Clarendon in April 1660, he declared 'a liberty to tender consciences'; and in a covering letter accompanying a copy of this document he assured the Speaker of the House of Commons, in a sentence of inordinate length and careful lack of precision, of his zeal for the Protestant religion. Not many people believed him, for he had been too long away and too infected by French contagion.

It is difficult for us today to comprehend the intensity of English feeling against Roman Catholicism at the moment of the Restoration. And it was this obsession which undermined Charles's relationship

with the various Parliaments of his reign. He himself was, if anything, a cheerful agnostic. He was also shrewd – or crafty – enough
to trim his sails to most of the prevailing winds. He contracted a
harmless marriage to the Catholic Princess of Braganza, but arguably
rather for the attractions of her dowry than for her physical qualities.
The spark which ignited the powder barrel was the conversion of
his brother James to the Catholic faith in 1668. Since Charles had no
legitimate heir, the succession would thus pass to the first Papist
monarch for over a century and this was anathema to the Parliamentary opposition. Charles had no affection for his brother (in this he
was not alone), but he held unshakeably to his belief in the hereditary
principle of kingship and in James's divine right of succession. For
thirteen years he conducted a running engagement with a hostile
Parliament dominated by two ruthless and implacable men, Shaftesbury and Buckingham, both dedicated to the destruction of Popery
even at the risk of another civil war. Charles fought a skilful tactical
battle. Where necessary – as in the case of the two Test Acts which
disqualified from public office all who refused to accept the Anglican
Sacrament and deny the Church of Rome – he conceded a few yards
of his political trench-system. But when Parliament tried three times
to force upon him a Bill excluding James from the succession in
favour of his eldest illegitimate son, the Duke of Monmouth, he
stood firm; and in Oxford, on March 28, 1681, he won the day.
Henceforth, he was monarch of all he surveyed and the last years of
his life were passed in an atmosphere of autumnal calm. And to the
end, he was short of money.

Out of these battles of the middle years, two things emerged
which were to change profoundly the face of political life in England. The first was the birth, as yet in embryonic form, of the party
system in Parliament – originally on the broad lines of 'Country'and
'Court' factions, but soon to be known as Whigs and Tories. The
second – and it is perhaps the most important of Charles's contributions to the progress of statecraft – was the development of a form
of constitutional monarchy which has survived, *mutatis mutandis*, to
the present day. Thereafter – and because, rather than in spite of,
James II's subsequent assault upon reason and moderation – the
sovereignty of Parliament was assured.

The years of religious skirmishing were to find a curious echo at
the Royal Hospital. The second Test Act had purged the army of all
Catholic officers, and since regimental commanders were their own
recruiting officers, they operated an unofficial test throughout the
lower ranks. The earliest surviving nominal roll of army pensioners

is dated February 1691 (one year before the Hospital eventually opened) and contains 562 names, including four Germans, eight Dutchmen and three exiled Huguenots (no whiff of Popery there!). At the end of the roll, as an anonymous afterthought, are added 'eight old Roman Catholicks at 4*d*. a day.' It was worth a penny more to be a Protestant.

While King and Commons indulged in their private power game, the people began to pick up the old threads of daily life which had largely been severed during the years of the Republic.

England at the Restoration was a predominantly agricultural country with a population of five and a half million (a quarter of Louis XIV's France and not significantly greater than the Dutch Republic). Then, as now, the people were independent, pugnacious, good-humoured, given to indolence, intolerant of foreigners, amenable to lawful authority, resentful of officious government. They have changed a good deal less than the country in which they lived.

That country was dominated by London where half a million souls were crowded along the north bank of the river between Wapping and Westminster. Piccadilly was open country and Islington, Knightsbridge and Chelsea, rural villages. Already the City was the commercial heart of the capital and Whitehall, with its sprawling palace, the seat of government. The river, crossed by a single bridge, was London's High Street, a busy thoroughfare linking the shipyards of the lower reaches with the farms and orchards of our modern suburbia. Even by the middle of the seventeenth century the English had become a nation of shopkeepers and Charles, who was quick to understand the temper of his people, once wrote to his sister, Minette, in Paris: 'The thing which is nearest the heart of this nation is trade and all that belongs to it.' By the middle of the century London was the centre of a growing colonial empire and the struggle for commercial and maritime supremacy was to be the mainspring of Charles's foreign policy.

This city was the wonder of the world, a curious blend of beauty and brutality, of serenity and violence. The London mob had long been notorious, respecters neither of rank nor person and ready to ride whatever political or religious whirlwind happened to be the fashion of the hour. It was to escape the attentions of Shaftesbury's 'brisk boys' that Charles retired to Oxford in 1681, there to summon (and dissolve) his last Parliament.

But London was not England. In the shires and counties the old squirearchy was still the order of the day and echoes from 'the great hive' were no more than distant reminders that high matters of state were being conducted there behind closed doors. After the capital, Bristol and Norwich were the largest cities, each numbering around 30,000 inhabitants. Birmingham and Manchester were still a straggle of villages set in a green countryside. Life proceeded at the pace of the plough. And despite great extremes of wealth and poverty, people lived well.

It was a country of good trenchermen and great tipplers, and while Charles's court, with its strong French influence, wined and dined with taste and discrimination, the people at large preferred quantity to quality. The Excise returns for 1685 give an output of 11,000,000 barrels of beer which represents an annual consumption of *72 gallons* per head of population and this takes no account of the substantial output – and intake – of home-brewed ale and west country cider. Beer cost ½*d.* a quart (no self-respecting Englishman would have contemplated the idea of pint measures) and by modern standards it was heady stuff. Eating was on the same scale. Middle-class Samuel Pepys entertained half a dozen friends to a dish of marrow-bones, a leg of mutton, a loin of veal, a plate of pullets and larks, a large tart, a neat's tongue, a dish of anchovies, and another of prawns and cheese, while the more elaborate tables of the nobility groaned under a staggering weight of dishes, cooked with an insular indifference to flavour or digestion. Menfolk convention-ally remained covered at table and an engraving of the Great Hall at Chelsea a hundred years later shows the pensioners wearing their cocked hats as they sat 'in good and decent order' at dinner.

While private soldiers, for the most part billeted on inn-keepers, fared indifferently (most of them in any case preferred a liquid diet), the common seamen subsisted on a basic ration of two pounds of salt beef and a gallon of beer a day. In due course, the In-Pensioners of the Royal Hospital were to be royally served. The first Instruction Book of the Hospital goes to extraordinary lengths to define the quality and quantity of their 'dyett' and the pensioners were enter-tained at a standard far above anything they could have afforded outside. They lacked for nothing except money, and money meant beer. Thus, with their old-soldierly instinct for a good thing, they established a brisk market in surplus rations with the local citizenry, and the surrounding taverns flourished exceedingly.

If the English may be said to take their pleasures sadly, that was certainly not true of Restoration England. Wine, women and horses were the ruling passions of the day and all were pursued with a singular lack of inhibition. London offered a wide range of entertainment; for the man in the street, the brutalities of the cock-pit and the bear-ring, and for the upper crust, the new sophistications of the stage. By 1662, two public theatres had been licensed in Drury Lane and Lincoln's Inn Fields, while the Court Theatre in Whitehall catered for the cosmopolitan tastes of Charles's own circle. At first the productions of the day were dull imitations of the French classical drama, but presently – as a natural reaction from Puritan morality – there emerged a new, very English style of comedy ranging from the saucy to the frankly pornographic. After the tight-lipped years, the English began to laugh at themselves again. Nonetheless, not every prospect pleased. On November 26, 1661, Evelyn noted: 'I saw *Hamlet, Prince of Denmark*, played; but now the old plays began to disgust this refined age, since his Majesty's being so long abroad.'

Outside London, the people of the countryside resumed their old pursuits and pastimes. It was a dangerous world for wild animals for they were enthusiastically pursued on horseback and on foot and the surviving game-books of the great country houses record a mighty slaughter of innocents. While the yeoman coursed for hares, the gentry chased the fox and the nobility hunted stags across their broad acres. Wild-fowling was a popular pastime, and on the banks of the Hertfordshire Lea, a contemplative gentleman had lately composed the first classic book of instruction on angling. There was dancing on village greens and traditional sports and games at the great seasons of the year, while travellers from across the border brought word of a new and curious game called 'goffe'. All England was at play.

But there was also work to be done. Already the English genius for cloth-making had established an universal renown – the broad-cloths of the West Country, drugget and serge, medley and baize, kerseys from the woollen looms of Yorkshire, Norfolk worsteds, and later the cotton fabrics of Lancashire. Farming occupied nearly half the population and the rapid growth of the enclosure system resulted in a striking increase in agricultural productivity. But it was also a nation of craftsmen working in leather and pottery, ironware and glass, hat-making and hosiery; and already particular industries were being established in those areas where they are still thriving today.

33

But above all, England lived by the sea and as the colonial empire grew and prospered, so the ports of the southern and western seaboards prospered too. Through these ports flowed the wealth of the Orient, and from Africa, America, and the West Indies came sugar and oil, tobacco and spices, and the newly fashionable tea and coffee. And from these ports sailed the ships of stout English oak carrying the products of English craftsmen and a new breed of merchant adventurers in search of rich new horizons.

There was little unemployment except where old industries were dying and the land was poor. A labourer's wage averaged 7*d.* a day 'without dyett' or 3½*d.* a day with modest food and drink. An artisan or a craftsman could earn £50 a year, an army officer £100. Further up the scale a lawyer's annual income might be as much as £200 (times have not changed), and a prosperous merchant's £500 when trade was good. Throughout the period, except during the two Dutch Wars, prices and the cost of living remained remarkably stable, particularly in respect of food; for it was a self-contained island, producing in abundance all that was required and importing only those luxuries which graced the tables of the court and the nobility – a thriving land poised on the brink of a great and growing prosperity. Before those calm waters were reached, there were still storms to be weathered, but the Restoration years mark the emergence of England as a new and significant world power and for this the King was largely responsible.

What manner of man was the 'pious' founder of the Royal Hospital?

Quot homines, tot sententiae. Of no king is this more true. The range of modern opinion extends from Arthur Bryant's romantic and warmly affectionate view, to the distaste – even contempt – of Maurice Ashley and George Clark. In between these opposite poles of black and white is every shade of grey and here perhaps the truest and fairest portrait of this unusual man lies in Dr Kenyon's witty, critical, but always charitable study.* Winston Churchill permitted himself no such charitable sentiments. He liked his heroes to have been officers and gentlemen, and in his eyes Charles II was neither. His own liberal Puritanism was repelled by Charles's elastic morals,

* See also David Ogg's *England in the reign of Charles II* (O.U.P.).

and his final, dismissive summing-up of this anti-hero is less than just and a good deal less than accurate:

> 'Apart from hereditary monarchy, there was not much in which Charles believed in this world or another. He wanted to be King, as was his right, and have a pleasant life. He was cynical rather than cruel, and indifferent rather than tolerant. His care for the Royal Navy is his chief claim upon the gratitude of his countryman.'

The In-Pensioners of Chelsea, among many others, have good cause to think otherwise.

No man knew Charles better than Chiffinch, his charmingly named personal servant and confidante, who was at his side from the years of exile until his death. But Chiffinch was the soul of discretion and committed nothing to paper. All that has come down to us are his detailed accounts of the King's expenditure of Louis XIV's frequent subsidies and these, in their own way, tell us that his master was an honourable man.

Many other contemporaries have left a record of their impressions of Charles and even his political opponents, with the single exception of Shaftesbury, found his personality irresistible. Evelyn's view of the man is suspect, for he was an arch-namedropper and obsequious in the presence of the great and famous. Thus the sour comments in his diary after the King's death are partly a reflection of his distaste for Charles's private life-style but more probably an expression of pique because, for all his worthy service, he had never received any preferment. But among those who had no particular axe to grind – men like Ailesbury, Bruce, Roger North and Sir John Reresby – there is only admiration or even affection, And so it was with the public at large.

The traditional image of Charles is that of the 'merry monarch', a label which he would have enjoyed. His court circle was notorious for its riotous life-style and the King himself set a lively pace. Six principal mistresses and fourteen accredited bastard children was a notable tally even by Restoration standards, and a source of much embarrassment to Catherine of Braganza who presented her randy husband with Tangier, Bombay and £500,000, but no Protestant heir and successor. Yet in his last hours this essentially kindly man sent to ask her forgiveness, even if his final thought was for Nelly, his 'Protestant whore', that she should not starve. Nor did she.

The man in the street readily identified with this merry monarch and held him in that special affection which the English reserve for an aristocratic 'card'. The nobility and gentry were less enchanted and the sanctimonious Evelyn could never resist a priggish broadside at the royal 'concubines'. A walk with the King in St James's Park in March, 1671 ended a little unexpectedly:

> 'Thence to the garden, where I both saw and heard a very familiar discourse between (the King) and Mrs Nelly, as they called an impudent comedian . . . I was heartily sorry at this scene. Thence the King walked to the Duchess of Cleveland, another lady of pleasure, and curse of our nation.'

Charles kept a strict dividing line between business and pleasure and his assorted ladies were firmly excluded from affairs of state; nor were they a charge upon the public purse. At least his vices were both natural and public, which is more than can be said of the later Stuarts. His brother James was privately no less promiscuous, while both William and Queen Anne cultivated homosexual liaisons. Of all this, for his peace of mind and tender conscience, John Evelyn was fortunately unaware.

The warrant for his arrest after the battle of Worcester in 1651 described Charles as 'a tall, dark man, six foot two inches high'. There was more of his grandfather, Henri IV, than of his father in his heavy features, and the harsh experiences of his youth and early manhood made him appear prematurely old. With his splendid physique, he excelled at all forms of sport and country pursuits, rising early to play tennis or ride by way of the King's Private Road to watch the progress of Wren's restoration of Hampton Court. He was a superb horseman and this was not to be wondered at for his teacher had been the old Duke of Newcastle, the foremost master of equitation of his day. With this – unusually – he combined a passion for the sea, and in fair weather or foul he would sail down river in the royal yacht to visit the busy shipyards on either bank of the Thames, or farther afield to Chatham or Portsmouth.

Of all the kings of England he was the most approachable and easy-going and he delighted to take exercise in St James's Park, walking with his long stride, his spaniels at his heels, stopping to feed the ducks or to talk to passers-by on every subject under the sun. He was a great talker and a witty one, though the prim Halifax had this to say of his conversation: 'His wit was better suited to his condition before he was restored than afterwards. The wit of a gentleman and that of a crowned head ought to be two different things.'

Above all, Charles loved Newmarket, and he would go there in the Autumn to escape briefly from the London scene and from his talkative and ill-tempered Commons. There he felt at home in the company of his friends and of the jockeys whose earthy humour matched his own. He was closely interested in bloodstock breeding, even if the names of some of the horses – 'Jack-come-tickle-Me' and 'Sweetest-when-Naked' – were rather less than kingly; and twice he himself rode the winner of the Newmarket Plate. When, towards the end of his life, the little town was burned down, he transferred his affections to Winchester where Wren was building him a palace and where he could divide his time between hawking and visiting his fleet in nearby Portsmouth.

He was a man of many parts and his legacy to the nation was an enduring one. Apart from the Royal Hospital, he established by Charter the Royal Society, the Royal African Company and the Hudson's Bay Company. He created the Regular Army and revived and greatly strengthened the Royal Navy. He rebuilt the City of London after the Fire. He founded the National Stud and introduced the first ducks and pelicans to St James's Park. Everywhere he planted trees and yet more trees. He was fascinated by the world of science, tinkering away happily in his private laboratory and putting Evelyn to work on a study of smoke pollution in London. His hand is still everywhere to be seen.

In every sphere the achievements of other men reflected his inquisitive and liberal mind. For this was the age of *Paradise Lost* and *Pilgrim's Progress*; of Dryden and Purcell; of Wren and Tompion. But above all it was the age of experiment and curiosity. The Royal Society, with its emphasis on the inquiring mind, drew together men like Newton, Boyle, Hooke, Petty, Halley and Evelyn. Outside that circle were medical pioneers like Sydenham and Wiseman and the great political philosophers Hobbes and Locke.

It was a golden age of the creative spirit, unequalled by any similar period in our history. How it might have developed if Charles had survived to old age is something on which we can only speculate. One thing, however, is certain. If, by an accident of history, Charles's brother, James, had ascended the throne at the Restoration, the country would very soon have been plunged into another civil war more bitter and bloody than that which Charles I had precipitated. James's combination of arrogance, stupidity and bigoted Catholicism would at that moment have destroyed the whole fabric of English life and it is impossible to tell what course the history of these islands might then have taken. The most likely outcome would have been invasion and occupation by the armies of France. And, quite certainly, there would have been no Royal Hospital as we know it today.

Whatever may have been the sins of omission and commission of Charles II (and they were many), his feeling for public relations was sure and accurate. He understood that the English people, emerging from the shadows, wanted colour and gaiety and he led them into the sunlight. He restored to them their sense of humour and their instinct for adventure, for this was the restoration of much more than just an ancient monarchy. He led them by example – not always too creditable – and he steered a middle course between the demands of an unruly Parliament and his own conviction of royal prerogative. He could be devious and dishonest, but rarely uncharitable, and inconsiderate only to those who presumed too much on his good nature. The twenty-five years of his reign provided, as it were, safe conduct for the English people from the prison which Cromwell had built around them, so that when in due course James succeeded him, the old passions had been damped down and the inevitable Revolution, when it came, was bloodless. That, with all deference to Winston Churchill, is his chief claim upon the gratitude of his countrymen.

Towards the end of his life a celebrated and anonymous verse went the rounds:

> *We have a pretty witty King*
> *whose word no man relies on.*
> *He never said a foolish thing*
> *and never did a wise one.*

Such *lèse-majesté* would not have amused Queen Victoria. It says much for Charles that his comment was entirely in character: 'That is very true, for my words are my own, my actions are my ministers'.'

Such, then, was the climate of the time and the nature of the man who set in train 'so exelent a worke' at Chelsea. Sadly, he never lived to see Wren's noble realization of the royal intent of which he had informed Sir Stephen Fox in the autumn of 1681. Charles would have loved the place. He, so relaxed among his Newmarket jockeys

___

and so accessible to the humblest of his subjects, would have enjoyed the company of his old soldiers whose bawdy language was on his own level and whose capacity for strong drink matched his own. Who were those old soldiers, how did they come to be in the King's service and what brought them in due course to Chelsea?

3
The King's army
❧

At Cromwell's death in 1658, the strength of the New Model Army was of the order of 40,000 men, with foot and horse in the proportion of two to one. In the short space of thirteen years, it had been tempered into the finest military instrument the country had ever known or was ever to know again until the 'contemptible little army' took the field in 1914; but now the sword was beginning to rust in the scabbard and the army which had been Cromwell's pride was feared and hated by the people; more fatally, it had begun to play politics.

The origin of the New Model Army goes back to 1642. Cromwell's first taste of battle on a large scale had been at Edgehill. There he had learned his lesson, as a troop commander of Essex's horse, that cavalry, properly trained and resolutely led, could and would be the decisive factor in the war. But first he needed men of indomitable spirit and determination.

Now in October he set to work with a troop of sixty men. By March of the following year the single troop had become a regiment of five troops and by September this had grown to ten. By the end of the year, its strength was fourteen troops numbering eleven hundred men. But it was quality, not quantity, that Cromwell sought. 'A few honest men,' he said, 'are better than numbers'. And by that he meant men who believed passionately in their cause and were prepared if necessary to die for it. He looked, too, for men of intelligence, for they would have much to learn and wars are not won by bravery alone. His regiment was an élite body and as such he subjected it to a rigid standard of discipline. God-fearing as he was, he expected no less from his officers and men. In return, he laboured to ensure that they were well-mounted, well-fed, well-equipped – and well-paid. Only in the last regard did he have less than absolute control. But within the year he had produced a regiment the like of which the country had never seen before. It was to prove itself conclusively at Marston Moor.

Yet one regiment was not enough. The quality and spirit which Cromwell had created there needed to be reproduced throughout the whole parliamentary army, if decisive victory was to be achieved.

So, as the war dragged on into 1645, the making of the New Model Army began. Its nucleus, not surprisingly, was Cromwell's old regiment, now divided into two under his cousin Edward Whalley and Sir Thomas Fairfax. Since it was to be available for general service this army was to be paid – and *regularly* paid – out of national funds. It must be dressed 'uniformly' – hence arose a new word and hence, too, came the scarlet coats which the British soldier was to wear for two and a half centuries and which today survive proudly at Chelsea. In short, this army was to want for nothing that would enhance its military spirit and its efficiency.

The New Model legislation, which was passed on February 13, 1645, laid down a strength of 22,000 – eleven regiments of horse, twelve regiments of foot, one thousand dragoons, and an artillery train; and to achieve these numbers conscription was introduced. Fairfax was appointed commander-in-chief with the rank of captain-general, Phillip Skippon commanded the infantry as major-general, and the appointment of lieutenant-general commanding the cavalry was left vacant – though not for long. In June, Cromwell was literally back in the saddle and at Naseby the New Model Army won the decisive victory which finally broke the Royalist forces in the field.

This army was an instrument designed for war. With the execution of the King in 1649, it found itself in the unaccustomed climate of peace, and in that climate it began to display a growing arrogance towards the people and towards parliament. When occasion arose, as in the battles of Dunbar and Worcester and in the battle of the Dunes, it proved that the old fires still burned strongly, even though its conduct in the Irish campaign remains a stain upon its honour.

When, at Cromwell's death, his ineffective son, Richard, was proclaimed Lord Protector, the army under Lambert presently made its bid for power. Once again the country stood on the brink of civil war. But the people had had enough of bloodshed – and more than enough of military dictatorship. They turned now to George Monk, the parliamentary commander in Scotland and himself a former Royalist. On February 3, 1660, Monk reached London. He restored the Rump Parliament which Lambert had dismissed the previous October; and amid scenes of extraordinary rejoicing, the King was proclaimed at Westminster and in the City on May 8.

We may pause here to consider the consequences of the New Model Army. Far from setting a future standard of efficiency or creating a sense of national pride, Cromwell's army left behind it a deep-rooted and ineradicable suspicion of military authority throughout the land. It is fair to say that, as a result, the Army has never since been popular except at times of national emergency or under the influence of a spurious jingoism. Curiously enough it reached perhaps its lowest point in public regard in the middle of the last century, at the height of Victoria's imperial noontide, and there are several In-Pensioners at Chelsea today who can recall notices in public-houses before the 1914 War which said bluntly, NO DOGS: NO SOLDIERS – in that order. The public attitude to the Royal Navy was always different, partly because sailors are less ubiquitous and partly because the Fleet was seen to be our island shield and guardian of the high seas on which our imperial greatness depended. Mindful of the Interregnum, Parliament kept a firm hand on the army and echoes of this running battle between soldiers and politicians recur throughout the history of the Royal Hospital. That it survived is a matter partly of luck and partly of conscience.

One of the first acts of the Restoration Parliament was to set in train the disbandment of the New Model Army. At the same time provision had to be made to meet the cost of this army (£55,000 a month) and the back pay of both officers and men which had fallen considerably in arrears since Cromwell's death. It is important here to draw attention to this aspect of public finance. From the time of the Restoration and for a century and a half afterwards, payment on due date was the exception rather than the rule; and this cavalier attitude applied no less to many private transactions. Throughout his reign, most members of Charles II's court were permanently in arrears – or were never paid at all. The same situation applied to army pensions after their introduction in 1685, though here, as we shall see, there was an official jackdaw at work. Many of the bills due to sub-contractors and craftsmen engaged in building the Royal Hospital were not met for as much as eight years. And even the Chelsea Board followed the practice of the day. A Board Minute in 1749 calmly observes that no window tax had been paid for *seven years* and proposes that a remittance on account would be a wise precaution. One glance at the Royal Hospital suggests that the outstanding sum must have been substantial, for the building then contained 712 windows.

Disbandment of the army proceeded by lot and would have been completed by the Spring of 1661, but for a sudden – and, as it proved, fortuitous – event. On January 6, a fanatic named Venner sparked off an insurrection of the eccentric Fifth Monarchy sect in the City of London. It was a minor affair which was quickly suppressed, but it brought Charles hurrying back from Portsmouth. More significantly, it provided him with the opportunity to halt the process of disbandment. He moved fast, for on February 14, General Monk's Regiment of Coldstreamers laid down its arms symbolically on Tower Hill and took them up again as the Lord-General's Regiment of Foot Guards. It was thus the only descendant of Cromwell's infantry and survives today as the Coldstream Guards.

So, almost by chance, the Regular Army came into existence. Its nucleus, apart from Monk's Coldstreamers, was drawn from those Royalists who had gone into exile with the King in France and Flanders: the King's Troop and the Duke of York's Troop of Horse which duly became the 1st and 2nd Life Guards; the King's Royal Regiment of Guards, which became the Grenadier Guards; and a newly-raised Regiment, the Earl of Oxford's Troop (the Blues), later to become the Royal Horse Guards.

Parliament looked suspiciously at this new development and refused to vote any supply for what it considered – at least to salve its conscience – as the King's private bodyguard. Nor at this stage did it attempt to obstruct the royal will when Charles embodied four more regiments in his standing army. Two of these had been for some years in the service of foreign powers: the 1st Foot (Royal Scots) in France as the Régiment d'Hebron, and the 3rd Foot (the Buffs) under the Dutch Republic as the Holland Regiment. They were embodied respectively in 1662 and 1665. Finally, after the King's marriage to Catharine of Braganza and the dowry of Tangier which accompanied her to the altar, two more regiments were formed: the Tangier Horse (1st Royal Dragoons) and the Tangier Foot (the Queen's Royal Regiment).

For most of his reign the King's army never exceeded 7,000 men except in 1678 when, under pressure of demand from Parliament for war with France, the numbers rose to 16,000. Yet curiously, in view of its pathological distrust of standing armies, one of the first decisions of the new Cavalier Parliament which met in May, 1661 was to pass a Militia Act which vested supreme control of the Militia, the Standing Army and the Navy in the Crown. It seems a strange conflict of interest. So far as the Militia was concerned, people could sleep peacefully in their beds. It was an ineffective body raised locally by persons with a minimum property qualification and controlled by Lords Lieutenant. All its members were required to attend a General Muster once a year and to spend not more than eight days in training. When mustered, they were paid at the munificent rate of 1*s.* a day for foot-soldiers and 2*s.* 6*d.* a day for troopers (the precise rates of pay of Cromwell's army). The infantryman's rate, allowing for changes in money values, was *fifteen* times that at which their Regular counterparts went to war in 1914. Not that this helped. The only time the Militia was called upon to put its training to the test was at the battle of Sedgemoor in 1685, where its conduct was so deplorable and its loyalty so suspect that it provided James II with an incontrovertible case for doubling the size of the Regular Army.

Such was the military situation as the Restoration began to move into troubled waters. And it is at this point that the mainstream of the standing army and the future tributary of the Royal Hospital begin to flow together – in the person of Stephen Fox.

Stephen Fox, a man of modest origins, was born at Farley in Wiltshire in 1627. At the age of thirteen, he obtained a position as Closet-Keeper to Prince Charles whom he followed into exile on the death of the King. There he appears to have been the general factotum at Court for, as Evelyn tells us, 'both the King and Lords about him frequently employed him about their affairs; trusted him both with receiving and paying the little mony they had.' His shrewdness – and honesty – were duly rewarded, for on the King's return to England, he was promoted from Clerk of the Kitchen to that of the Green Cloth, a post which gave full scope to his financial acumen; and in 1661 he was appointed the first Paymaster-General of the Forces.

He was to serve the Crown through four reigns and his philanthropic acts extended far beyond the Royal Hospital. These included a large contribution to the rebuilding of the College of Arms after the Great Fire and to repairing the nave of Salisbury Cathedral. In 1678 – prophetic touch – he founded an almshouse, designed by

Wren, at Farley for six old men and six old women, together with a chapel and a school for six boys and six girls. In 1693 he built Farley Church, also to Wren's design, and two years later some almshouses at Broome in Suffolk and at Castle Ashby. He must have been a remarkable man for he amassed great wealth at an early age by his own honest endeavours, and that, in Restoration England, was a very singular achievement. He was knighted in 1665.

As Paymaster he received £400 a year for himself and his clerks together with a deduction of 2*d*. in the pound from Army pay to cover Exchequer fees. As we have seen, the King's revenue was entirely inadequate (in any case Parliament relegated the standing army to the lowest priority) and so, in keeping with the spirit of the times, soldiers' pay soon fell into arrears. The troops were not slow to voice their complaints to Monk, now Duke of Albemarle and Captain-General, and Fox came to the rescue. He undertook to pay the army punctually on a weekly basis and raised the necessary money by pledging his own credit. Here his reputation had preceded him so that, as Evelyn tells us, 'he obtained such credit among the banquers that he was in a short time able to borrow vast sums of them upon any exigence' – which was more than the King could do.

But for all his philanthropy, Stephen Fox was first and foremost a businessman and he had his price. Samuel Pepys, in his diary entry for January 16, 1667, explains:

'Sir Stephen Fox told me his whole mystery in the business of the interest he pays as treasurer for the army. They give him 12*d*. per pound quite through the army, with condition to be paid weekly. This he undertakes for his own credit, and to be paid by the King every four months. If the King pay him not at the end of every four months, then, for all the time he stays longer, my lord treasurer allows him by agreement eight per cent per annum for the forebearance. So that, in fine, he hath about 12 per cent. from the King and the army, for fifteen or sixteen months interest, out of which he gains soundly, his expense being about £130,000 per annum.'

This arrangement appears to have been popular with the troops, on the principle that nineteen-twentieths of a loaf is better than no bread. Fox continued this system of payment with the King's tacit approval for eighteen years when, on his appointment as a Treasury Commissioner, he asked to be relieved of his responsibilities for army pay 'by reason of the difficulties of the revenue'. It is interesting to note that at this date the establishment of 'all our Guards, Garrisons and Land Forces in this our Kingdom of England' totalled 6,872 at an annual cost of £203,954 9s. 5¼d. The King accordingly issued a royal warrant recognizing 'the absolute necessity of constant and steady payment of the troops' and directing that in return for regular payment the deduction of 12d. in the pound should be continued. And Fox continued to draw one third of the poundage fund until the end of 1683, by when, according to Evelyn, 'he is believed to be worth at least £200,000, honestly gotten and unenvied, which is next to a miracle.'

This poundage fund is very relevant to our story for, as we shall presently see, it was to provide the main source from which the building and financing of the Royal Hospital was maintained for the next hundred years. And to that extent the army may be said to have paid for its own veterans' home.

The establishment of the King's army was, as we have seen, on a very modest scale and its ranks were filled from those gentlemen (the definition is important) who had followed Charles into exile; and from old soldiers, Cavalier and Roundhead, most of whom were experienced veterans. All engagements were on a permanent basis which meant in theory that a man signed on for life; and this in turn created a new situation – and a new problem.

Under the old feudal system of private and semi-private armies the responsibility for maimed and worn-out soldiers rested with each man's captain or 'overlord'. Such men were normally lodged in the various hospitals set up by monastic orders or wealthy benefactors, but in pre-Tudor times there is no reference to any system of pension or compensation for disability or long service. With the dissolution of the monasteries and 'the going away of hospital lands and revenues' the situation had become critical and a complaint had been made to Lord Burghley regarding 'disfurnishing the realm of places to send maimed soldiers to' and 'enfeebling their hearts when they know not how to be provided for if they are maimed.'

Eventually, in 1593, an attempt was made to devise a statutory provision for disabled soldiers. This took the form of a measure entitled 'An Acte for reliefe of Soldiours' which directed that men

46

who had 'adventured their lives or lost their limbs in the service of Her Majesty and the State should at their return be relieved and rewarded. . . . that they may reap the fruit of their good deservings . . .'

The reward took the form of weekly rates not to exceed 6*d.* nor be less than 1*d.* in the pound to be levied in parishes and to be distributed in the form of pensions payable quarterly at a maximum rate of £10 a year for ordinary soldiers. It was in theory a worthy and charitable object – if it had worked in practice. But local authorities either ignored or evaded the terms of the act, and this resulted in a flood of petitions to the Crown. The Domestic State Papers of Queen Elizabeth are peppered with these and they appear to have been largely effective. The earliest instance, in 1595, is 'a grant to Edward Lloyd of a pension of 12*d.* a day for life' (no mean sum at that date), while in the following year there is the first recorded case of 'a grant to William Evans, a maimed soldier, of an alms-room in Durham.'

The Act of 1593 was renewed twice by Elizabeth and again by James I. It continued to be honoured more in the breach than in the observance. And there were some wily customers around. Thus a certain William Wyatt petitioned the King for relief as a maimed soldier from the county of Oxford pleading the King's promise to him at Woodstock: 'Thou shalt not be wronged.' His claim was submitted for verification to the local Justices who duly reported that the said William Wyatt 'has no certificate to prove his being a maimed soldier, on the contrary he has lived in the county as a labourer for twenty years.'

The case of Hugh Drayton of Atherstone was different, but has a not unfamiliar ring: 'October 23, 1620. The said Drayton did revile the King in his drink for nonpayment of his pension of £16 a year. Indorsed with a note that he is penitent and is to be whipped or otherwise corrected. Petition from inhabitants that a little drink distempers his brain, and makes him speak improperly. He is occasionally *non compos mentis* from wounds in the war.' Drayton was duly whipped, reinstated as a pensioner – and died a month later, presumably 'in his drink'.

It was from this period that the first modest 'hospitals' for old soldiers date. The earliest is that founded in 1571 for twelve 'decay'd and decrepid' soldiers by the Earl of Leicester at Warwick and shortly afterwards Thomas Sutton accommodated some forty old men in the Charterhouse. Perhaps the most interesting of the early institutions is the Coningsby Hospital at Hereford, founded in 1614 for a company of eleven – 'one Corporall and ten old Servitors, six of the Servitors to be oulde souldiers of three years service at least in the warres. . . .' While it is a far cry from Coningsby to Chelsea, there are a number of significant points of detail. The old men were dressed in semi-military uniform – 'a fustian suit of ginger-colour, a hat with border of white and red, a soldier-like jerkyn . . . and a soldier-like sword.' The corporal received 3*s*. 4*d*. a week and the servitors 2*s*. 6*d*. The company was remarkably well fed and the 'dyett' included the inevitable 'two full quarts of beer each day, one at eleven o'clock and the other at six o'clock'. Sir Thomas Coningsby was himself an old soldier and wise to soldiers' ways, and his regulations laid down strict penalties for any of his company 'who haunts tavernes or aleshouses or is a common Drunkard, quareller, brabler or who lives incontinentlie or who is proved to beg or cosen. . . .'

In spite of these acts of private charity the problem of old, sick and maimed soldiers remained intractable. The Civil War served only to underline the problem, and for the first time funds were raised not from the local rates but from 'sequestration money' – a primitive step towards a national pension fund. Indeed, in 1651 the Commons went so far as to consider the possibility of erecting 'a healthful place for such decayed souldiers' residence.' However, more pressing matters of state intervened and the idea does not appear to have been pursued; and thus, at the Restoration, the care and sustenance of old and disabled men was still largely a matter of private benevolence or local charity.

It must soon have become clear to Charles II that the existence of a standing army would eventually require some formal and permanent arrangement for the welfare of disabled or superannuated soldiers. In the early years of his reign the problem was not a pressing one since, with the exception of the Tangier garrison which was administered under local arrangements, the army was not involved in active service (the two Dutch wars were almost entirely naval affairs), and the newly embodied regiments could only date their period of service from 1661 at the earliest. There still remained, however, a considerable body of Civil War veterans and of Royalist supporters who had been financially ruined under the Commonwealth and these men were not slow to voice their grievances to the

King in writing or, to his greater embarrassment, in person whenever he walked abroad in public. Many of these letters have been preserved and perhaps the most remarkable is one addressed to the King in June 1666 by an anonymous lady whose indignation is equalled only by her illiteracy. She launches into the attack at once: 'I am extremly grived to heare the sad condishion this kingdom is now in.' She continues briskly with some sharp comments about the tax burden – 'This makes a great crie amunst the comon people; they curs the King and wish for Crumwell' – and then turns her attention to the conduct of the royal courtiers, the royal concubines, even the royal personage himself. 'Your nation finds that you car not what becoms of them, soe you have your pleasure; you think not of the sighs and grons your poor subjects uter, but I doubt they will not be subjects long, their pacienc hath binn upon ye tenter houks a great while.' Then she comes to the heart of the matter; the treatment of the King's soldiers. And here her angry outburst contains more than a grain of truth: 'It is reported that your Ma'ty should say there is nothing lik keeping the soulders poore. . . . If Your Maj'ty did but heare the slits and scofes that is mad; for, saie the people, be a soulder, noe, we have presedents daily in the streets, we will fight no more, for when the wars is over, we are slited lik dogs [*a phrase which Kipling was to echo two centuries later*].'

Charles must have smiled when he read this broadside, but the very fact that the letter has survived suggests that he took its central message seriously. He was already at odds with Parliament and could ill afford any dissatisfaction in the army. Unfortunately he could equally ill afford the cost of that army.

A possible solution shortly presented itself across the Channel, where the problem of providing for old soldiers of the French army had long exercised successive monarchs. No legislation existed for this purpose in France and attempts by Henri IV and Louis XIII to establish military hospitals had both foundered for lack of funds. Thus wounded and superannuated men – *les stropiats*, as they were known – found such care and sustenance as they could in monastic institutions, while the State divested itself of all responsibility for them.

With the massive expansion of the French army under Louis XIV, some formal system of State aid had become imperative and by an ordinance of February 24, 1670, the King gave instructions for the foundation of a Hospital 'for the support and succour of soldiers wounded or disabled in war or who by virtue of their age are incapable of continuing in His Majesty's service, such soldiers to be fed, clothed and entertained in an Hôtel which His Majesty is causing to have built for this purpose'; and on April 15, the foundation was formally named the *Hôtel Royal des Invalides.*

The money for this elaborate project was raised by confiscating the pensions of *les oblats*, the lay monks of the various religious orders, who for the most part were themselves old soldiers. Half the funds thus raised were devoted to the building of the Hospital and the other half to the provision of pensions for infantry officers. And on March 12, 1670, a Royal Warrant directed that the sum of two deniers in the livre out of ordinary and extraordinary monies provided for the prosecution of the wars should be set aside for the maintenance of the new institution.

Under the terms of the foundation, entry was originally restricted to Catholic officers and other ranks, but was later extended to Protestant veterans. For some curious reason, artillerymen were at first refused admission to the Hospital despite the indignant protests of the Master Gunner, the Duc de Maine,* and it was not until 1716, after the King's death, that the ban was removed.

The *Hôtel des Invalides* was Louis XIV's especial pride. So much did he look upon it as his personal charity that he expressly forbade by law the making or acceptance of any outside donations towards its embellishment or upkeep. This direction has survived to the present day so that when, at his death in 1941, Alfonso XIII of Spain, the last lineal descendant of the *Roi Soleil*, left a substantial property in Rouen to the Hospital, the bequest was politely but firmly declined.

In his will, Louis expressed himself thus:

'Among the various institutions which we have established in the course of our reign, there is not one which is of greater value to the State than the *Hôtel Royal des Invalides*. It is right and proper that soldiers, who by reason of the wounds they have received in war or by virtue of their long service or their age are no longer

---

* When the Duc de Maine pressed Louis for his reasons for this discrimination, the King replied airily that he was 'répugnant aux nouveautés'!

able to work or earn their living, should be properly sustained for the rest of their days.'

and he enjoined his successors 'to support this institution and to accord it their personal and particular protection.'*

The Invalides was one of the very few royal institutions to be respected by the leaders of the Revolution – and with good reason; for the mob which stormed the Bastille armed itself by the simple expedient of raiding the armouries and powder-store of the Hospital.

The designer of the Invalides was Libéral Bruand, the Architect-Royal, who is remembered today solely by this monumental work. The site chosen was in open country on the left bank of the Seine and the King's instructions were simple and typical: a true *Maison Royale* on the largest scale, worthy of its lofty purpose and worthy of the resplendent city then rising across the river. The result is probably the purest example of Louis XIV style in the grand manner of that grandest of ages.

The north front presents an imposing façade flanked by two pavilions. A massive entrance leads into a spacious and cloistered Court of Honour, beautifully proportioned and built in a warm honey-coloured stone, on the far side of which stands the *Église des Soldats*, the heart of the Hospital and a reminder of the monastic origins of the foundation. On either side of the Court of Honour are four identical enclosed courtyards. The two on the left contained kitchens and refectories, and the infirmary and annexes leading to six small interior courts, each a single storey high and so designed as not to mask the later addition of the dome. To the right are two matching courtyards which contained the living quarters and refectories of the *invalides*, and beyond them the priests' lodgings and gardens. Some indication of the scale of Bruand's plan may be gauged from the fact that it was designed to accommodate up to 4,000 men (compared with Chelsea's 476).

The four main refectories each held 400 men, with two sittings for each meal, so that there was a capacity of 3,200 places at table. Meal times were punctiliously observed and any man parading even one minute late was ordered to return to his quarters by the armed guards stationed at each door, ostensibly to prevent the removal of

* After a visit to the Invalides, Montesquieu wrote: 'Had I been a prince, I would rather have founded this institution than have won three battles. Everywhere the hand of a great monarch is to be seen. I believe it to be the place most worthy of respect in the whole world.'

food after the meal. A 'delinquents' table' in each mess provided an exquisitely French touch, for here sat the *buveurs d'eau*, the old soldiers who had committed minor breaches of discipline and whose punishment was to be restricted to drinking water instead of the *invalides'* staple diet of wine.

A separate mess was set aside for senior ranks and, finally, one small refectory was reserved for blind pensioners who were treated with special care and consideration.

Bruand's plans were approved on March 15, 1671 and by May, 1673 the building was complete except for the roofing of the central section. The Hospital was formally opened on April 15, 1674 and by the end of the year the first 2,000 *invalides* had taken up residence.

At this point Bruand seems to have fallen foul of the Marquis de Louvois, Minister of War, for the design and construction of the great dome which is the distinguishing feature of the Hospital was entrusted to the celebrated Jules Hardouin Mansart. This dome, which surmounts the second church built as an extension to the *Église des Soldats* and which to-day contains the tomb of Napoleon, was consecrated on August 28, 1706. Apart from a small extension to the original structure on the south-west side in 1749, it was the last and crowning glory of Louis XIV's noble enterprise. The *Hôtel des Invalides* stands to-day unchanged across three centuries, though much of it is sadly marked by the passage of time.

The original ordinances did not stipulate a minimum age for admission but simply laid down as qualifications wounds sustained in action or ten years effective service in the army. Within a short time the Hospital was so inundated with applications that in 1709 it became necessary to close the entry lists, while the strain on financial resources was such that the 'poundage' levy was increased to three deniers in the livre. The following year the service qualification was increased to twenty years and admission granted only direct from regimental service, while officers of units raised during the War of Spanish Succession were only accepted into the Hospital in the rank of sergeant.

As the pressure of applications continued, a large number of old soldiers were lodged temporarily in the annexe of Gros-Caillou outside the Hospital walls, a step which added greatly to the cost and even more to the administrative confusion. To provide vacancies for urgent and deserving cases, men were sent outside to 'detached companies' (in much the same way that Companies of Invalids were used to create vacancies at Chelsea), and out-pensions were offered to those who agreed to withdraw their applications for entry.

Eventually in 1776 the Hospital establishment was reduced to 1,500 all ranks, at which date there were 6,000 *invalides* in detached companies and 18,000 Out-Pensioners in the provinces.

To-day the scene has changed radically. Libéral Bruand's great building has experienced a steady encroachment from outside. The Court of Honour now houses the superb *Musée de l'Armée*. The *Hôtel des Invalides* plays host to the Military Governor of Paris and to Army Inspectorates and military organizations of every description. Only the old Infirmary remains as the *Institution des Invalides*, and here there are 210 beds for permanently incapacitated patients, while old soldiers throughout France are entitled to claim admission for treatment on surrender of 30 per cent of their service pension.

Gone are the uniforms of the *Maison du Roi*. Gone is the old asylum behind its moated wall. Gone are the *buveurs d'eau*. The long refectories are filled with the panoply of distant wars. Yet though much is changed, the great institution which Louis XIV founded in 1670 remains to honour the soldiers of France.

The Invalides clearly created a great impression in London and Charles must have realized that a foundation on a similar, although smaller, scale was no less essential for the future well-being of his own old soldiers. But once again he found himself at loggerheads with the House of Commons. Early in 1679 Parliament had declared all military forces to be illegal, and in that political climate, the proposition of building a retreat for army veterans would have been an explosive issue; and financially Charles was in no position to proceed with such a plan in defiance of the Commons.

There remained, however, as a quite separate issue, the army of the Irish establishment which was accepted, albeit with ill grace, by the English Parliament as a necessary evil in a country largely compounded of necessary evils. By 1675 the strength of the army in Ireland stood at 7,000 men, described by their Marshal, the Earl of Granard, as 'becoming grey in ease and routine'. Since, however, no system of superannuation existed, no action was taken until the appointment in 1678 of the Duke of Ormonde as Lord Lieutenant.

Ormonde at once recognized that the Irish Army had not only become grey in ease and routine, but also so inefficient through age and decrepitude that it was incapable of any serious military activity.

He had also made a thorough study of the organization and administration of the Invalides. Thus in the summer of 1679 he set forth his proposals for the establishment of a military hospital at Kilmainham on the outskirts of Dublin and on October 27 he was authorized by letter by Charles to proceed, on the understanding that the project should not be a charge upon the Irish Exchequer.

Ormonde, perhaps the greatest public figure of his day, had served Charles for thirty years and had himself grown grey in the intricacies of royal finance. He had also inherited, predictably, in Ireland the inevitable situation by which army pay had fallen seriously into arrears, in a country whose total annual revenue amounted to a bare £300,000. He accordingly proceeded with some ingenuity. Through the good offices of two financiers, 'Robert and William Bridges, Gentlemen', he raised a loan of £36,500 to clear the soldiers' arrears. And this loan he in turn repaid by charging poundage of 1s. in the pound on the pay of all ranks. Thus over a period of eighteen months, the Irish Army unwittingly paid the debts due to it by anticipating its own future emoluments – a very *Irish* solution.

By March 29, 1679 the accounts had been brought into balance, and from that date the poundage rate was reduced to 6d., to be applied strictly 'as a provision for aged and infirm soldiers'. And from this reduced fund Kilmainham Hospital was built and financed.

The plans for the new hospital were drawn up by Sir William Robinson (not by Wren, as has commonly been supposed) and the foundation stone was laid by Ormonde on April 29, 1680. The building was completed in less than four years at a cost, including the land, of £23,559 16s. 11¼d. The original establishment specified 300 In-Pensioners, based on a wastage of thirty men a year, but the estimate proved no less inaccurate than that which we shall see in due course at Chelsea, and by 1685 provision had to be made for an Out-Pensioner element which grew progressively until by 1822 – when their administration was transferred to Chelsea – the total had risen to 15,379.

We need not concern ourselves here with the organization and administration of Kilmainham, for it was gradually adapted to correspond with that at Chelsea, even to details of dress and subsistence. But it is interesting to see how Irish veterans were entertained at table, in a country not then noted for its lavish standard of living. The first Instruction Book laid down the following diet at a cost of 1¾d. a day per man:

'*Monday*   Mutton and Broath
Tuesday   Mutton, Veale or Lamb, Roast
Wednesday   Pease and butter
Thursday   Beef, boyled
Friday   Fish as season requires
Saturday   Burgooe
Sunday   Beefe, Roast

Each man having a Pound of meat after drest, and over and above a sufficient allowance of Broath and Water Gruell and Stirabout. Each man to be also supplied 18 ozs of bread daily at rate of £5 per week for 217 men.'

The first Kilmainham In-Pensioners soon displayed the whimsical characteristics of their race. Within five years forty-seven had been dismissed from the hospital for persistent drunkenness, seven for 'causing affrays', seven for begging, while Pensioner Joseph Tully was 'sent out of the charity' for the curious crime of 'undoing the Chaplain'.

The Kilmainham poundage of 6*d*. ceased in 1794 and the establishment was maintained thereafter by Parliamentary votes. The first official attempt to close the hospital down occurred in 1834 and thereafter the In-Pensioner establishment was reduced to 200. A second unsuccessful attempt to close the hospital was made in 1853 and was followed by a further reduction in numbers to 140. There for the moment we will leave the old Irish veterans until they make their final appearance after the First World War. But Kilmainham was by no means their only home and they soon began to infiltrate the Long Wards at Chelsea where to the present day they have continued to dispense their native charm and bland disregard for authority in equal measure.

In March, 1681, Charles finally grasped the nettle and dissolved Parliament. It was not to meet again in his life-time, and now he was free to dispose of his adversaries in his own time and in his own way. He was also free to act upon those long-considered plans which a hostile Commons had been determined to frustrate. On September 1, Lord Longford, Master of the Ordnance in Ireland, attended upon him in Whitehall and gave him a full account of progress in the building of Kilmainham. There is no record of their conversations but on September 8, shortly before setting out for Newmarket, Charles gave verbal instructions to Sir Stephen Fox for the establishment of a similar hospital for the old soldiers of the English Army. And thus, almost casually, the great enterprise was set in train.

4
'Condidit Carolus Secundus'

❦

By the autumn of 1681, Sir Stephen Fox's circumstances had changed, for he was now a Treasury Commissioner. Five years earlier, for reasons of personal jealousy, he had been dismissed from the Pay Office by the then Lord Treasurer, the Earl of Danby, but with Danby's fall in 1679, he was appointed to the Treasury. From December that year, the office of Paymaster-General was held jointly by Nicholas Johnson and Fox's eldest son William who died a few months later, leaving Johnson in sole charge.

Stephen Fox was the obvious and natural choice to carry out the King's intention to build a hospital for his old soldiers. He was known and respected for his honesty (a rare virtue in men of affairs around Charles) and he was still responsible for financing army pay through his private credit. And since the dissolution of Parliament earlier in the year, the King had had no constitutional source of supply. Nonetheless the credit for founding the Royal Hospital has been the subject of much speculation and it is worth adding a little grist to the mill.

Tradition has long maintained that the idea originated with Nell Gwyn, even though modern historians, those most unromantic of men, have gone to great lengths to dismiss the story as legend. She was born in February, 1650, the daughter of a feckless Welsh army captain who had fought in the Royalist cause. Her birthplace is unknown but has been variously ascribed to Coal Yard Alley, a former slum behind Drury Lane; Oxford; and Hereford. If indeed it was Hereford, she may well have seen the old 'servitors' of Coningsby Hospital as a child. But it was in London that Evelyn's 'impudent comedian' was to make her mark, and even the attentions of the King, no less, did little to change her earthy nature or her bawdy wit. She learned with difficulty to write her initials on the only documents that mattered, her receipts 'for services rendered', and to her last day she remained virtually illiterate in all but her own special – and very professional – subject. She also had a nicely waspish sense of humour. When Charles asked her to choose a country house, she – mindful of her arch-rival, the Duchess of

Portsmouth, and her estate at Goodwood – picked as her own 'royal' residence *Best*wood Park near Nottingham.

The historians are probably right. Yet the fact remains that, of all Charles's mistresses, she was the only one of humble origins and it is not too fanciful to believe that the sight of old and crippled soldiers begging in the streets moved her to draw the King's attention to this melancholy situation. Among the In-Pensioners today, old traditions die hard. 'To think,' observed one wistfully, 'that we are all living in a royal brothel.'

More probably the idea originated from discussions between the King and Sir Stephen Fox. There is no record of any such conversations, but a later memorandum in Fox's hand is quite specific:

> 'This great Charity sprang from ye Innate goodnesse of his Sacred Majestie, who seeing old Land Soldiers, after having served in his Royal Guards & other of his Majestie's Land Forces, beg for not being able (by Age or infirmity) any longer to continue their duty, it so affected his Royall mercifull brest, that without any other motive, of himselfe was pleased to command that, Notwithstanding his then Nessessitous condition (Never Lower), an Hospitall should Immediately bee erected. . . .'

Noblesse oblige! Yet Fox's obeisance needs two correctives. At the end of 1681, the King's finances were in better shape than at any time previously in his reign; and the matter of motive is not quite so innocent. There can be little doubt that Charles was concerned at the plight of his old soldiers, for he was a compassionate man; but there was a more practical consideration. Twenty years had now passed since the formation of the standing army and relations between soldiers and civilians had become increasingly strained. Most of the troops were kept under canvas at Hounslow where distance lent some measure of enchantment. But the royal Guards billeted in and around Westminster and conducting themselves with an arrogance that recalled the worst days of the Protectorate, were both a public scandal and a social irritant. Indeed, as one contemporary recorded, 'to be a Guardsman is now accounted a very evil thing'.

As morale declined, so did the level of enlistment; and there can be no doubt that the real reason behind the Royal Hospital was to provide a stimulus to recruiting, a light at the end of the long tunnel of military service towards which old soldiers could wend their way. In their discussions the King and Sir Stephen Fox had obviously planned for a building which could accommodate the entire existing wastage in the army. They could not have foreseen that events would soon confound all their estimates.

Thus Fox gracefully attributed the foundation of 'this great Charity' solely to the King. But his was not the last word on the subject. In a sermon delivered at Fox's funeral in 1716, Canon Eyre had this to say:

> 'He [*Fox*] was the first projector of the noble design of Chelsea Hospital and contributed to the expense of it above £13,000 [*a slip of the tongue; the figure was £1,300*]; and his Motive to it I know from his own Words, he said, "he could not bear to see the Common Soldiers who had spent their strength in our Service to beg at our doors", and therefore did what he could to remove such a Scandal to the Kingdom.'

In less than a week after the King's departure for Newmarket, Fox set to work. On September 14, Evelyn recorded:

> 'Dined with Sir Stephen Fox, who propos'd to me the purchasing of Chelsey College, which His Majesty had some time since given to our Society, and would now purchase it againe to build an Hospital or Infirmary for Soldiers there, in which he desired my assistance as one of the Council of the R. Society.'

The choice of Chelsea as the site of the proposed Hospital was dictated by a number of factors. We do not know the various alternatives which Charles and Sir Stephen must have considered, although there is some evidence to show that they gave a good deal of thought to both Windsor and Hampton Court. But there were obvious reasons, both psychological and practical, for deciding on a location within easy reach of Westminster. And money was not the least of their considerations. Nonetheless, it was fortunate that they made the choice they did. Somehow one feels that posterity would not have taken too seriously the image of 'Tooting Pensioners' or 'Pimlico Pensioners'. Chelsea, perhaps fortuitously, sounded right and proved to be right.

In his diary entry of September 14, Evelyn refers to 'Chelsey College', and this requires a brief explanation. In 1609, James I had founded a theological college for the study of 'polemical divinity' on a piece of ground called 'Thames Shott', a 28 acre field which corresponds broadly to the area on which the present Hospital buildings stand, bounded on the north by Royal Hospital Road and on the east by Chelsea Barracks. In the best Stuart tradition, James's enthusiasm for anti-popery was not matched by available funds with which to finance the project. A poll-tax, to be paid on taking the oath of allegiance, produced a negligible revenue, an appeal to the Archbishops and clergy even less, and so far as we may judge such money as was forthcoming was provided by Matthew Sutcliffe, Dean of Exeter and the first Provost of the college. In the event the project was a fiasco and only a small part of the building was completed, on the site of the present South-West wing. During the Republic, this building was used to house Scottish and foreign prisoners of war. In 1665, it was handed over to the ubiquitous Evelyn in his capacity as Commissioner for the Sick, Wounded and Prisoners of the second Dutch War, when most of his charges fell victims to the Great Plague. Two years later Charles presented the College to the recently formed Royal Society 'as a gift of His Majesty, our Founder', subject to a ground rent of £2 7s. 4d. a year.

It proved to be a somewhat back-handed compliment, for the following year the roof collapsed and Sir Christopher Wren, himself a member of the Royal Society, proposed that the dilapidated building should be pulled down forthwith. Though Wren could not then have known, it was a prophetic suggestion.

Though not himself a member of the Royal Society, Sir Stephen Fox must have heard that the Council was anxious to dispose of its white elephant. Earlier in 1681, Wren had been elected President of the Society and since he was also the King's Surveyor-General of Works, this must have strengthened Fox's negotiating hand. In the event the Council of the Royal Society instructed Wren and Evelyn on October 5, 'to treat with Sir Stephen Fox about selling the house and the whole concerns of the college for £1,500 if it might be agreed, but not under £1,400.'

On his return from Newmarket Charles became deeply involved in the final legal confrontation with his old adversary, Shaftesbury, and the matter of Chelsea College seems to have been shelved. There was another reason. Lawrence Hyde, son of the old Earl of Clarendon and now First Lord of the Treasury, strongly disapproved of the King's proposal for a hospital for his old soldiers as an unnecessary and unwarranted extravagance, and forthwith refused to sanction any Exchequer support for the project. It was not the wisest of tactics, for Charles was no longer in any mood to tolerate obstructive ministers; and he was no stranger to financial stringency. Hyde's opposition must merely have strengthened his resolve.

The answer was provided by Sir Stephen Fox, for at this point he undertook to purchase the Chelsea College property out of his own pocket and convey it to the King. Thus the first hurdle was surmounted and on December 7 Charles issued his Royal Warrant, confirmed on December 22 by Letters Patent:

> 'We doe intend to erect an Hospital for the relief of such Land Souldiers as are, or shall be, old, lame, or infirm in ye service of the Crowne, and to endow the same with a Revenue suitable thereunto. . . .'

The Warrant continues by appointing 'Nicholas Johnson, Esq., the present Paymaster of Our Land Forces, and the Paymaster of our Land Forces for the time being, Receiver General and Treasurer of all such moneys as shall be from time to time given or paid for, or towards the erecting the said Hospitall, or the support or maintenance thereof during our pleasure.'

In these words the King founded his village in Chelsea. The problem of carrying out his instruction now fell to others.

On January 11, 1682 the Council of the Royal Society noted in their Minutes that the Chelsea College property had been sold to the King through Sir Stephen Fox 'for the building of an Hospitall' for the sum of £1,300 'ready money', and they proceeded to record a vote of thanks to Sir Christopher Wren for services rendered. Fox had made a good bargain, for the price was a most modest one, even by the standards of the period. He now had a site.

He next needed a plan and a design. Above all, he needed money.

On January 27, he invited Evelyn to dinner. 'This evening Sir Stephen Fox acquainted me againe with His Majesty's resolution of proceeding in the erection of a Royal Hospital for emerited souldiers on that spot of ground which the Royal Society had sold to his Majesty for £1,300 and that he would settle £5,000 per ann. on it, and build to the value of £20,000 for the releife and reception of four companies, namely, 400 men, to be as in a Colledge or monasterie. I was therefore desir'd by Sir Stephen (who had not only the whole managing of this but was, as I perceived, himselfe to be a grand benefactor, as well it became him who had gotten so vast an estate by the souldiers) to assist him, and consult what method to cast it in, as to the government. So in his study we arranged the Governor, chaplaine, steward, housekeeper, chirurgeon, cook, butler, gardener, porter, and other officers, with their several salaries and entertainments. I would needes have a Library, and mentioned several books, since some souldiers might possibly be studious, when they were at leisure to recollect. Thus we made the first calculations, and set downe our thoughts to be consider'd and digested better, to show his Majesty and the Archbishop. He also engag'd me to consider of what laws and orders were fit for the Government, which was to be in every respect as strict as in any religious convent.'

It is a charming picture – these two English worthies seated after dinner over their port, and planning the first details of a foundation that would survive them across three centuries. Neither Fox nor Evelyn – nor indeed the third of the triumvirate, Wren, who would shortly add his expertise to theirs – were versed in military affairs; and yet it is a remarkable fact that their original proposals needed very little amendment by the time the building was ready for occupation, and indeed remain the basis of the Hospital's organization and administration today. Since they had no domestic model, it is interesting to note Evelyn's references to a 'monasterie' and a 'religious convent'. It was, in their view, to be an almshouse on an entirely novel scale and to it they therefore applied the only disciplines they understood.

Stephen Fox now transcribed the notes they had made that evening and produced the following draft establishment, based one may assume, on a wastage of about 5 per cent of the mustered strength of the army:

> '4 Companys consisting of
> in all – 384 Private Sentinells
> 8 Drummers
> 12 Corporalls
> 8 Sergeants
> 4 Ensigns
> 4 Lieutenants
> 1 Martiall and Adjutant
> 1 Governor
> being 422 military persons'

all entered at their army rates of pay.

To these were added an administrative staff – 'Chaplain, Phisitian, Apothecary, Brewer, Butler, etc.' – of twenty-nine persons. The estimated cost was put in at £5,578 a year for 'military persons', £1,075 a year for 'ye usefull persons', and running costs, which charmingly included 'Nessessarys and Utensils for ye Garden', at a further and very precise £1,095 12s. 11d. a year. In a marginal note Fox indicated the cost of an In-Pensioner's diet at 6d. a day which, even allowing for price differentials, was lavish indeed compared with the 1¾d. a day at Kilmainham.

When ten years later the Hospital opened with Wren's extensions completed, the actual establishment was:

26 'Captains' (ex-Guardsmen)   @ 3s. 6d. a week
34 Light Horse (ex-Cavalrymen) @ 2s. 0d. a week
32 Sergeants   @ 2s. 0d. a week
48 Corporals and Drummers   @ 10d. a week
336 Private Men   @ 8d. a week

a total of 476 In-Pensioners, with an administrative staff of thirty-seven men and twenty-six women. And the ration allowance was 3½d. per man, per day. Only in terms of In-Pensioners' pay (or 'peculiar money' as Fox called it) had he set his sights too high, but it must be remembered that the out-pension scales were not laid down until 1685 and thus he had no comparable yardstick. In the event the total cost of running the Royal Hospital in its first full year amounted to £8,831 6s. 2d.

Armed with these preliminary estimates Fox now turned to the design of the Hospital itself. He did not need to look far.

Christopher Wren was born at East Knoyle in 1632, and thus, by a strange coincidence, both the chief 'architects' of the Royal Hospital happened to be Wiltshiremen. He first made his mark at Oxford, not in the arts but as a scientist, and Evelyn who met him at All Souls referred to him as 'that miracle of youth'. His talents ranged widely over the fields of astronomy, mathematics and physics and thus it was a curious, though inspired, choice when in 1662 the King appointed him deputy to Sir John Denham, the Surveyor-General of Works. Wren's services were soon in demand for in 1663 he was commissioned to design the Sheldonian Theatre in Oxford, an astonishing achievement for a man who had never yet set his

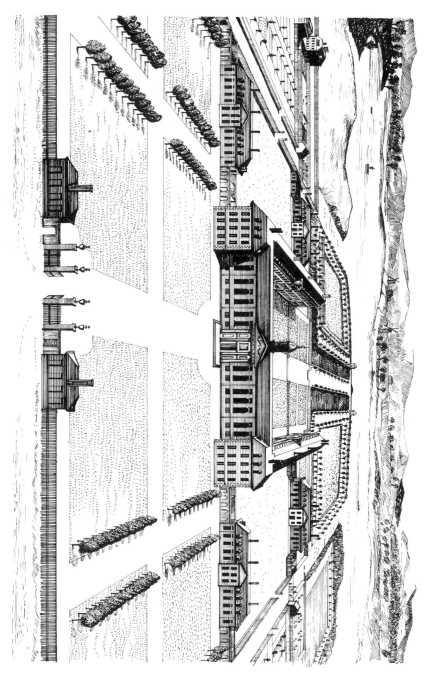

The Royal Hospital, c. 1690, after an engraving by J. Kip

hand to architecture, but who now mastered an intricate problem of construction by a mixture of instinct and geometrical expertise.

But instinct and geometry were not enough and two years later Wren paid a visit to Paris. It was the only occasion in his long and busy life when he travelled abroad, and he used the ten months of his stay to good advantage, studying the new architectural glories of the Sun King's capital. There he learnt and absorbed the technical rudiments of his trade, but throughout his life he was to be an innovator and only in the unfinished palace which he designed for Charles at Winchester and, to a lesser degree, at Chelsea can one detect any markedly French influence.

Shortly after his return, in 1666, there occurred an event which was to dominate the rest of his life. The Great Fire of London destroyed virtually the entire City and although still only deputy to the Surveyor, Wren was appointed to the Commission charged with its rebuilding. In particular, the new St Paul's Cathedral was to occupy him for over thirty-five years, but within the first half of that period he also designed or re-designed no fewer than fifty-two City churches, quite apart from numerous secular commissions. It is a measure of this extraordinary man's capacity for work that during the ten years which it took to build the Royal Hospital (and quite apart from his many commitments in the City), he also built or designed St James's, Piccadilly, Winchester Palace, the new White-hall Palace, the William and Mary buildings at Hampton Court, and Kensington Palace.

With Isaac Newton he was incomparably the greatest figure of his age, a simple, dedicated craftsman of whom John Flamsteed, the first Astronomer Royal for whom Wren had built the Royal Observatory at Greenwich, could write: 'He is a very sincere honest man: I find him so, and perhaps the only honest person I have to deal with.'

There is no record of Wren's formal appointment as architect of the Royal Hospital, but since he had become Surveyor-General in 1669, we may assume that a royal commission such as this was automatically his responsibility. It was, in any case, a challenge which must have greatly attracted him. Hitherto nearly all his work had been concentrated in the ecclesiastical field or on new or re-designed additions to university colleges; and all had been in an urban setting. Now for the first time he had an opportunity to create a major complex of buildings welded into an architectural whole and in a setting which allowed him a space and freedom previously denied him by cramped city streets or by the need to harmonize his own designs with those of other, earlier hands. It was a magnificent opportunity.

The Royal Hospital is the only major work of Wren's for which no drawings have survived. Their disappearance has never been explained and it seems particularly strange in the light of the meticulous care with which he preserved not only the finished designs but also the rough sketches for all his other buildings. There is one naughty possibility. For seventeen years, from 1685 to 1702, Wren served as a Commissioner of the Hospital with Stephen Fox and the Earl of Ranelagh, Paymaster-General throughout that period. Ranelagh, as we shall see, was a rogue in the classic mould and, among other misdemeanours, not only lined his pocket out of Chelsea funds, but also built himself an elegant residence in the grounds. It would certainly have served his purpose to arrange for Wren's original drawings to be 'mislaid' for they would have provided material evidence of his fraudulent activities. And it would have been quite in keeping with the character of a man who, when challenged by a committee of the House of Commons to produce the Chelsea accounts for the period *1688 to 1702*, flatly refused to do so.

Nonetheless there has survived among Sir Stephen Fox's papers a detailed description of the original building plan, and with the benefit of hindsight we can trace the progress of Wren's concept of the Hospital.

Fox's notes had proposed an establishment of 422 'military persons' and twenty-nine 'usefull persons'. Thus Wren knew the size of the problem. Fox and Evelyn had also indicated that the occupants of the Hospital were 'to be as in a College or monasterie'. Thus Wren worked on the premise that his design must be based on a unified requirement – a communal home where men could eat and sleep and worship. But they were not ordinary men. They were, in the words of Charles's Warrant 'old, lame or infirm in ye service of the Crowne', and carefully and often touchingly Wren took account of this fact.

Unlike existing almshouses, this was to be a *royal* Hospital and therefore it must have a suitable and monumental dignity. But it was not a royal *residence* and therefore, with wise restraint, Wren designed a building of great simplicity without excessive ornament or

66

sovereign flourishes. The King's old soldiers should have the best;
but they did not need – or expect – a Versailles.

There was another reason. Charles's Warrant had said: 'We doe
intend. . . . to endow the same with a Revenue suitable thereunto. . . .'. It was a fine, bold sentiment, but Fox must have warned
Wren at the outset that this grand enterprise was being launched on
something less than a shoestring. Wren would not have been surprised. After all, he had been a member of the St Paul's Cathedral
Commission for seven years and knew all about silk purses and
sows' ears. But as he studied the site, with its surrounding fields and
the meadows running down to the river, his mind must have gone
back to some of the French palaces he had seen, set in their elegant,
ornamental parks, and he decided upon a similar setting for his
Hospital, with buildings and gardens designed as a single architectural unit; and for this he needed more land.

We need not concern ourselves here with the complex details of
land acquisition which have resulted in the present Royal Hospital
property, but we may summarize the main features as they affect the
original Wren design. Between the Hospital site and the river lay
some 29 acres of meadow and these were conveyed to the Crown by
their owners, Lord Cheyne, William Green and Sir Thomas
Grosvenor between the years 1682 and 1686, and during this period
the Hospital also acquired from Lord Cheyne the strip of land on its
western boundary on which Gordon House and the National Army
Museum now stand. Finally, in 1687, Lord Cheyne sold the 13
acres of Burton's Court which lay on the north side of the old road
from Westminster to Chelsea.* With these acquisitions, Wren's
grand design was complete.

We may ask why Wren, on his tight and fragile budget, pressed
for so great an acreage of land. To explain this is to demonstrate the
grandeur of his vision and the quality of his mind. When, in January
1682, he stood on the site of Chelsea College, he was surrounded by
open fields – arable and pasture land and riverside meadows. Away
to his right lay a small cluster of houses, the village of Chelsea. The
rest was green and fertile countryside. His aesthetic instinct must at
once have rejected the idea of a monumental building set in the
middle of a great farmyard, and although he could not possibly have
foreseen the later growth of 'the Great Wen', he must have insisted

* The total cost of the original grounds was £5,079 16s. 6¼d. – no bad invest-
ment. It would be interesting to know what the value of the present Royal
Hospital property of 66 acres is worth today. An educated guess has put the
figure in excess of £120,000,000.

that his Hospital should be preserved from urban encroachment. That was his strictly practical view. His *architect's* eye envisaged a grand enclosure, approached from the north across the green space of Burton's Court and sweeping down to the river through formal, terraced gardens. It was one of the rare instances when he borrowed from his French experience and in so doing he created what must have been one of the great vistas of English architectural design. He was not to know that time and Victorian vandalism would destroy his splendid vision. What, one wonders, would he say today if he stood in Figure Court and looked across the river? Battersea power station he would probably appreciate as a kind of industrial 'cathedral', but he would be revolted, as others are, by the grey and graceless gas-holder nearby. And he would be angry, above all, if he could now see the destruction of his stately water garden below the South Terrace.

For his old soldiers' retreat, Wren experimented for the first time on a large scale with brick and stone under a grey slate roof. His choice was largely dictated by cost, but he was also concerned with the problems of colour contrast in a rural setting. The result is not entirely successful, particularly on the North Front where the effect is monotonous and where the panels above and below the tall windows, and the windows themselves, are picked out in a commonplace and brighter shade of brick. It cannot have been Wren's intention to leave these panels blank, but since his original drawings no longer exist, we can only assume what was in his mind. A few years later the Hospital accounts refer to an item for plasterwork in these panels, presumably as the base for some kind of mural decoration, but this was never completed and the plasterwork was later removed. When, in his maturity, Wren returned again to the marriage of brick and stone at Hampton Court, the result was to be perhaps the most beautiful and elegant of all his buildings; but at Hampton Court he was designing a royal palace, and William III was a man of continental taste and not short of money.

Wren's drawings for his original Hospital were completed by May 25, 1682, when he accompanied Fox and Evelyn to show them to the Archbishop of Canterbury for his approval. Evelyn, in his account of that visit, compares the building to 'the larger quadrangle at Christ Church, Oxford', but the two have nothing in common other than sheer size and Evelyn was probably only quoting 'Tom Quad' as a reference which the Archbishop would at once recognize. In fact Wren's design, to be known as Figure Court, was not a quadrangle, but a three-sided square, open to the south in order to

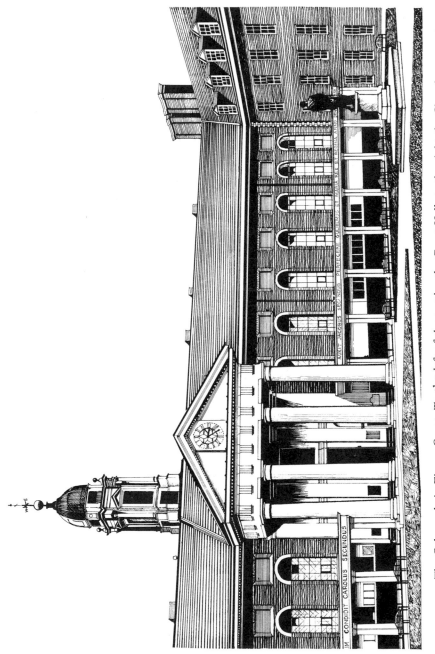

The Colonnade in Figure Court. To the left of the portico the Great Hall, to the right the Chapel give the maximum light and to provide a vista over the gardens and down to the river. The site presented him with problems. Its depth was restricted by the foundations of the old Chelsea College, the high road from Chelsea to Westminster, and the bank sloping down to the meadows and the river. He was accordingly compelled so to orient the building that it faced south-east with the result that half the In-Pensioners' wards get little direct sunlight. He must have pondered this problem carefully, for throughout the Hospital design the comfort and well-being of the old soldiers was his paramount concern.

Mindful of the 'collegiate' or 'monastic' concept of the Hospital, Wren centred his plan on a northern block consisting of the Great Hall and the Chapel, separated by a tall octagonal vestibule, or porch. Here was the communal heart of his Hospital; and here we find the first of his considerate touches, for the shallow steps ascending to the Hall and the Chapel are furnished on both sides with handrails for the old men. At either end of this block is a square 'pavilion' which contained, next the Great Hall, the kitchen and steward's quarters, and next the Chapel, 'the Infirmary and under it the Landery.' On the south side of this block, and broken by a massive portico of Portland stone, Wren designed a 'cloister' or colonnade with wooden benches running the full length of the wall on which, protected from wind and weather, the old soldiers could take the sun. And here, on the frieze above the colonnade, Wren set the Latin inscription which prefaces this book and which to this day informs the sole purpose and function of Charles's 'noble charity'.

From this central and communal block Wren then carried two great wings towards the south, each terminating in a 'pavilion' exactly matching those which flank the Great Hall and Chapel. Here were his 'collegiate' dormitories, the In-Pensioners' living quarters Stephen Fox thus described them:

> 'The two sides of ye Courte are double building in three stories and garrets, both containing 16 galleries [*or wards*], in each of which are 24 Cells divided off with partitions of Wanscot, and two larger Cells for corporals in each gallery, accommodating in all 416 single beds & each gallery hath two large chimnies and cisterns and conveniencys for water. 4 great staircases at both ends of each wing convey to all the galleries.'

Wren had catered almost exactly for Fox's original estimate, and it was not until the Long Wards were partly completed that it became evident that additional accommodation would be required.

Wren's design for the Long Wards is an interesting reflection of his intensely practical mind. Always considerate of the old men who would live there, he decided on separate cubicles, unlike Kilmainham and the Invalides where four or six men shared a ward. These cubicles were admittedly tiny – only six feet by six feet – but they provided an element of privacy which the old soldiers had probably never enjoyed before and which is a particular requirement of increasing years. Such personal belongings as the men possessed – and they were probably very few – were therefore kept in chests and presses in the corridors. And these corridors had also to serve as places of recreation and relaxation.

Wren therefore had two alternatives. Either he could place the cubicles against the outer walls, where they would get the best natural light, and leave a broad communal corridor to serve two wards; or he could set the cubicles back to back in the centre with two outside corridors. The first alternative, while probably the most natural, would have raised heating difficulties and it would also have meant that, deprived of natural light and in an age of flickering candles, the recreation facilities of the corridor would have ceased except during hours of full daylight. He therefore chose the form in which the Long Wards exist today. They must have seemed positively palatial to their first occupants; and few, if any, could have known the luxury of the bedding supplied – 'a straw mattress, flock mattress, bolster, feather pillow, two pairs of *linen* sheets, three blankets and a coverlet'. Between them, Fox and Wren set out to ensure only the best for the King's In-Pensioners. Finally, there remained the problem of access to the upper floors for old and often crippled men. Here the thoughtful Wren designed a series of staircases with broad, shallow steps and linked to an ingenious system of landings. The In-Pensioners would have to wait 250 years for the solace of electric lifts.

There remained the two pavilions at the southern end of each wing. The eastern pavilion contained – as it still does – the Governor's residence and the magnificent State Apartments. The western pavilion was designed to accommodate the officers of the house and today contains the quarters of the Lieutenant-Governor and the Adjutant.

In this fashion Wren began his grand design. On August 4, 1682, Evelyn 'went with Sir Stephen Fox to survey the foundations of the Royal Hospital begun at Chelsey'. Work proceeded slowly owing, no doubt, to lack of funds. A week before his death on February 6, 1685, Charles came to inspect progress. By then the main fabric of the Great Hall, the Chapel, the Vestibule, the entire West and part of the East wing had been completed, though the glazing, plastering and wainscotting had not been started. The King, it seems, was delighted with what he saw, yet four more years were to pass before the building was ready for occupation. Why the old soldiers were then kept waiting another three years before they could take up residence is one of many mischiefs which can be laid at the door of the first Earl of Ranelagh.

The expenditure on the 'Charles II' buildings amounted to some £50,000, or in other words rather more than twice Sir Christopher Wren's original estimate. This is accordingly a convenient point at which to summarize the arrangements for financing the building of the Royal Hospital.

With his gift of £1,300 for the purchase of the Chelsea College property, Sir Stephen Fox had set the ball rolling. On Christmas Day, 1681, Charles had given 'about £2,000 out of his more particular private mony in his own Hands, to begin so exelent a worke.' This was, in fact, a payment on account, for the King subsequently increased the sum to £6,787 4s. 2½d. which represented 'the ballance of money which was in his hands for Our secret service'. The effect upon 'Our secret service' is not recorded.

Here, at any rate, was a modest fund of some £8,000, enough on which to launch the project. Charles now turned to the fund-raiser's conventional stand-by, a public subscription; and on February 16, 1682, accompanied by a well-chosen retinue of dignitaries, he laid the foundation stone. This was anticipating events with a vengeance, for Wren had scarcely begun his ground-plan, let alone his architect's drawings, nor has the first stone ever been located. It was, in fact, a simple exercise in public relations, for four days later the *Domestick Intelligence* announced:

'Since his Majesty has been pleased to lay the first Stone of the Foundation of the Colledge to be erected for the maimed and decayed Officers and Souldiers, several of the Nobility have done the like, and contributed largely towards the carrying on so charitable a work.'

And a month later, the paper published another, similar announcement.

Unfortunately, both statements were some way short of the truth. Apart from the King and Sir Stephen Fox, precisely *eight* persons contributed out of their own pockets. This lukewarm response is the clearest possible evidence of the public antipathy towards the King's army. And the contributors, who deserve a better memorial than the Royal Hospital has conceded them today, were predictably men in or around the royal circle. Here they are, with a note of their individual contributions:

*Tobias Rustat,** Page of the Back Stairs	£1,000	0	0
Sir Leoline Jenkins, Secretary of State	£100	0	0
Thomas Tuston, later Earl of Thanet	£500	0	0
William, Earl of Craven, Colonel, Coldstream Guards	£20	0	0
William Blathwayt, Secretary-at-War	£241	10	0
Dr *William Sancroft*, Archbishop of Canterbury	£1,000	0	0
Executors of the *Bishop of Winchester*	£500	0	0
Executors of *William Mortimer, Esq*, Merchant	£200	0	0
	£3,561	10	0

With interest on this sum, together with that on the King's donation, the royal and public contributions amounted to the princely sum of £12,907 11*s.* 4*d.*

This scarcely represented the King's idea of 'a Revenue suitable thereunto', so Charles dug a little deeper. He instructed Fox to address himself to the Archbishops of Canterbury and York, soliciting contributions from the clergy, though why the cloth should have been expected to support the military is not immediately clear. Ebor was certainly not amused and wrote petulantly to Cantuar, disassociating himself from the royal round-robin with the words: 'Hatred & contempt we may get, but noe money.' The idea was quietly dropped.

By the end of 1682, the building fund for the Hospital had not reached even half its target and nothing had been raised towards the

---

* Rustat also commissioned Grinling Gibbons, for a fee of £500, to make the statue of Charles II, improbably dressed as a Roman General, which stands to-day in Figure Court. It was erected there by William III in 1690.

eventual maintenance of the Pensioners or the upkeep of the establishment. Charles therefore had recourse once again to the ingenuity – and generosity – of Sir Stephen Fox. Fox no doubt was aware that the Invalides had been built and endowed by deductions of pay from the French army. He also knew that the Duke of Ormonde had employed a similar device to pay off the arrears of the Irish establishment. Here, then, lay at least part of the solution.

In April of that year, Fox's second son, Charles, had succeeded to the Pay Office on the death of Nicholas Johnson. It was a very convenient appointment since it meant that, through his son, Stephen Fox could keep control of the Hospital project without becoming involved in day-to-day detail. And he was still drawing his pound of flesh for underwriting the soldiers' pay. It was to this source that the King now turned. On May 17, 1683, Letters of Privy Seal were issued allocating one third of the poundage fund to the Royal Hospital and back-dated to January 1, 1681. The sum involved amounted to £10,000, and since it came out of Stephen Fox's pocket, we may assume that it was a voluntary act of charity on his part. More importantly, it represented the first permanent source of revenue for the Hospital and one which could – and would – grow as the size of the standing army increased.

But it was still not enough; and on March 17, 1684, a Royal Warrant was issued increasing the poundage allocation from one-third to two-thirds, calculated to produce about £6,700 a year. Fox must have realized at this point that since the public would not support the Royal Hospital, the army – for whom it was designed – would have to do so. His logic – primitive but effective – was that of the contributory pension fund, and he now came up with two variations on the same theme.

The first was the deduction of one day's pay per annum (two days in a leap year!) from every officer and man in the army. This was authorized by a Royal Warrant dated June 17, 1684, but for some reason the stoppage was not enforced until the following reign, when the sharp rise in the strength of the army virtually doubled the revenue for which Fox had budgeted. The men in the ranks must have begun to wonder at what point *they* would be paying the *Paymaster.*

The second variation was short-lived and unproductive, and consisted of a levy of 12*d.* in the pound on both the buyer and seller of army commissions. It was introduced in March 1684, and discontinued nine months later when Charles withdrew his consent to the practice. In the event, it produced a little over £1,300, largely because Regimental Colonels contrived to get exemption on the very dubious grounds that they already had considerable financial commitments in running their units. Since, in fact, no Colonel worth his salt made less than £1,000 a year out of army contractors, one can understand what was meant by 'commitments'. At this date, the officer strength of the army was 251, with an additional ninety-three stationed in the various garrisons; and the records tell us that an ensign's commission was worth between £200 and £300, a lieutenant's about £400, while on two occasions a captain's commission changed hands for the astonishing sum of £3,000 (about £45,000 at today's going rate).

Fox had now established, by one means or another, a permanent source of revenue for the Royal Hospital – provided that the money was correctly and properly applied. In later chapters we shall see that this money was indeed to prove the root of considerable evil; but this the honest Stephen Fox could not have foreseen.

The poundage fund and what came to be called 'day's pay' continued to be the main source out of which both the Royal Hospital and all Out-Pensioners were financed and paid until Edmund Burke's Pay Office Act of 1783. The intervening hundred years will provide us not only with some ripe examples of man's inhumanity to man, but also of the standards of public conduct in the eighteenth century. *Condidit Carolus Secundus.* He little knew what he had started.

5

'Auxit Jacobus Secundus'

❧

With the death of Charles II, both Wren and Stephen Fox must have viewed the situation at Chelsea with some anxiety. The main building was far from completed and the present and future endowment still insufficient for the furthering and maintenance of the great project. Moreover, by the end of the previous year, it had become clear to Fox that he and Evelyn had got their sums wrong. Already the number of old soldiers qualified for admission to the Hospital was in excess of the original estimate of '422 military persons' and Charles's Warrant had pre-supposed that *all* his 'old, lame or infirm Land Souldiers' should be accommodated at Chelsea. In January, 1685, Wren had, in fact, already started to sketch out a plan for extending his original design. On February 6 the King died.

Wren and Fox could have had no illusions about his successor. Even if they had not met him personally (and both of them must have done), they could have been in no doubt about his reputation. In almost no respect – other than his promiscuity – did James resemble his elder brother. Stubborn, arrogant, absurdly – and at times dangerously – inarticulate, he was obsessed with his passion for the Catholic faith. Thanks to Charles, he had survived every attempt of his enemies to exclude him from the succession, but having arrived at his rightful inheritance, he ignored the danger signals and eventually destroyed himself. Yet unlike Charles, he was a man of action. Lord High Admiral during the Dutch wars, and a brave and experienced soldier, he was also, unlike many men of action, a capable administrator. Probably to the surprise of Wren and Fox, he was to prove in his short reign a lively and powerful advocate of the Royal Hospital, yet by a curious irony, he also contributed, through one disastrous decision, to the corruption and mismanagement which was to bedevil the Hospital for over a hundred years and more than once bring it to the point of extinction.

Upon his accession, James addressed the Privy Council thus: 'I have often heretofore ventured my life in defence of this nation; and I shall go so far as any man in preserving it in all its just rights and liberties.' The Privy Council was delighted. It was also very naïve. James's speech-writer – he was incapable of composing so

succinct a statement of policy himself – had struck a properly
Delphic note. Phrases like 'just rights and liberties' are capable of
various shades of interpretation.

James had assumed that, upon his succession, he would be faced
with the prospect of either sporadic or organized rebellion. He
knew instinctively that he could rely upon his brother's standing
army in the way that all professionals rely upon each other. To his
surprise he now found that the English people can be very unpredictable. When, in May, 1685, he summoned his first Parliament –
the first, in point of time, since Charles had dismissed the Commons
at Oxford four years earlier – he found himself confronted with an
overwhelming Royalist majority. Not for the first time, and certainly not for the last, James misread the signs. The people had
accepted his protestations of political and religious freedom. They
had mistaken licence for liberty.

When James met his new Parliament, he told them, with a curtness
that his brother would never have ventured, that he required an
adequate and sufficient supply with which to conduct the affairs of
state. A dutiful Commons accordingly voted him a sum for life
almost twice that which they had ever conceded to Charles, including an annual £800,000 for the Navy and – for the first time –
provision for 'the maintenance of the royal guards and garrisons'.
Stephen Fox must have raised an eyebrow at this.

But before the gossips could get to work, something happened
which was to transform not only the political scene, but also the
future of the Royal Hospital. In the middle of May, the Duke of
Monmouth, eldest of Charles II's illegitimate sons, sailed from
Holland with 150 supporters and on June 11 landed at Lyme Regis.
He had come, he announced, as Charles's legitimate heir and
therefore as rightful successor to the throne, and would submit his
claim to a free parliament which would replace the unlawful assembly
recently summoned by James.

There was no immediate rush to join his standard but within a
fortnight he had raised a rebel army of some 500 horse and 4,000
foot, ill-equipped and with few experienced officers, but sufficient
to cause the local militia to take to the woods. At the head of this
motley force of irregulars, Monmouth campaigned in leisurely
fashion through the West country as far as the gates of Bristol
where for the first time he met organized resistance. There he
paused.

After the initial panic had subsided in London, James dispatched
a regular contingent consisting principally of the seasoned regiments

of the Tangier garrison which had returned to England two years previously, and at the night battle of Sedgemoor, near Bridgewater, on July 5, they inflicted a crushing defeat on the rebels. Monmouth was captured and executed, and the infamous Judge Jeffreys seized the opportunity to conduct his 'campaign in the West' against all those who had supported the rebellion.

Monmouth had unwittingly played a trump card for the King. Any doubts or inhibitions that James may have entertained were now laid aside. The conduct of the militia in the field and the danger to the realm of any similar acts of aggression from outside gave him irrefutable grounds for increasing the size of the standing army, and on the evidence available Parliament could scarcely obstruct the royal will. By the end of 1685, the strength of the English establishment had risen to around 20,000 by the raising of seven new regiments of horse (in due course to become the seven regiments of Dragoon Guards), the Scots Guards, and nine regiments of infantry (the 7th to the 15th regiments of foot or, by modern title, the Royal Fusiliers, King's Liverpool, Royal Norfolk, Royal Lincolnshire, Devonshire, Suffolk, Somerset Light Infantry, West Yorkshire, and East Yorkshire). By the middle of 1688, this number had been further increased by the addition of two regiments of Dragoons and five of infantry.

James now had the bit firmly between his teeth and his romanizing zeal took charge. Without recourse to Parliament, he dispensed with the first Test Act and appointed Roman Catholics to high offices of state and other key positions; he followed this up by similar appointments to commissions in the army. This latter action, while certainly in defiance of the law, was also a matter of practical necessity. The rapid expansion of the army had created a serious shortage of officers and James could hardly be expected to ignore the large reservoir of experienced men who had been put on the shelf by the Test Acts and whose only crime was their religious conviction. It may also be asked how the King was able to recruit so many rank and file for his new army when the principle of military service had fallen so low in public esteem. The chief answer is that there is nothing like an invasion – even an abortive one – for closing a nation's ranks and attracting men to the colours. But James, who was as shrewd as he was stubborn, had another card up his sleeve; and this he was to play within three weeks of Monmouth's defeat at Sedgemoor.

On November 19, however, James addressed the new session of Parliament and informed the house that the militia had been shown to be ineffective in a national emergency and that 'a well-disciplined standing force was indispensable to guard against all disturbances from without and from within'. And he added injury to insult by admitting that he had appointed to commissions officers who had not taken the test.

Parliament was dismayed, for it found itself hoist with its own petard. It therefore offered the King a substantial grant of £700,000 provided he would use this money to reform the militia as an alternative to the standing army. However, the arrogant and self-confident James was in no mood to bargain. He rejected the proffered grant and in the best Stuart tradition prorogued Parliament on November 30. Although it was not dissolved until July 12, 1687, it never met again during his reign. By this wilful action, the King had sown the seeds of his own destruction; and never again was an English monarch to be permitted to rule without Parliament.*

Meanwhile, shortage of money had brought progress to a virtual halt at Chelsea. Early in 1685, James had renewed the allocation of two-thirds of the poundage fund for the purposes of the Hospital and later in the year he put into practice the stoppage of a day's pay throughout the army which his brother had earlier approved by Royal Warrant. The continuing expansion of the army now ensured an increasing revenue from these two sources. Many years later, Sir Stephen Fox recorded that 'there was then a deduction of about £12,000 p.ann. out of the Army for the said Hospitall', which made possible the establishment 'for the maintenance of about 500 soldiers, besides the Officers & everything relating to the Hospitall.'

Even while Monmouth was manoeuvring in the West country, two more sources of revenue for the Royal Hospital were tapped. On June 4, at the proposal of Sir Christopher Wren, the House of Commons voted to apply part of the proceeds from licensing hackney coaches 'to Chelsea Colledge'. This seems to have been implemented for only one year during which time it produced around £2,000. However, so many hands were dipped into the till that eventually little more than £700 reached the Hospital Treasurer. And since by then that post was occupied by the Earl of Ranelagh, this remaining sum vanished without trace, a fact which was not discovered until

---

* Constitutional purists may point to the Prince Regent's arbitrary dissolution of 1818.

nearly twenty years later, by which time Ranelagh was insolvent and the money beyond recovery.*

Finally on June 16, the King obtained from the corporation of Newcastle-upon-Tyne an annual endowment of 100 chaldrons (about 60 tons) of coal in return for the surrender of certain royal property leased to that corporation. This arrangement continued until 1807 when the Crown property in Newcastle was sold and subsequently the contract was commuted for an annuity of £173, which in turn continued until 1872, when it was terminated on Treasury instructions.

James from the outset took a lively interest in the Royal Hospital, for it accorded closely with his own ideas for rewarding long and faithful service to the Crown. He often visited the old soldiers billeted around the town and awaiting entry into the Hospital, and while this was largely an exercise in public relations, there was another, more characteristic, reason. The Rev. G. R. Gleig, a nineteenth century Chaplain of the Hospital and a prolific, if inaccurate, chronicler of its early history, tells this pleasant, though probably apocryphal, story:

'James is said to have paid frequent visits to the hospital and to the veterans awaiting admission in and around the area, appealing first to one and then to another of the veterans to return within the pale of the Church of Rome; until a fine old warrior on a certain occasion cut him short in a manner which he could neither forgive nor resent.

'"Why should you not adopt the religion of your prince?" said James. "Please, your majesty," was the reply, "I was once a Catholic; I then became a Protestant; and I should be very happy to go back to your majesty's religion again, only when I was in Tangier, I entered into an agreement that the next time I changed my creed, I should become a Turk."'

James must have been particularly irked by the fact that Wren was building a Protestant chapel at Chelsea, but here, at least, he was wise enough not to abuse the royal prerogative. The fact that the superb chapel plate, made in 1687 and 1688 by Ralph Leete and bought from John Rogers for £542 8s., bears James's cypher does not mean that he either knew of or authorized the purchase. And we may imagine that when eventually, in 1963, a Roman Catholic

* Every summer the London Taxi Drivers' Benevolent Association take a party of infirm Pensioners on an outing to Brighton. Although they may not know it, they are repaying in kind the cash that never came to Chelsea!

chapel was consecrated in Sir John Vanbrugh's beautiful eighteenth-century Orangery, the ghost of this most humourless man must have contrived a small, wry smile of satisfaction.

Wren's sixteen 'gallaries', or wards, in the East and West wings had been designed to accommodate 416 men, including sergeants and corporals. Fox now realized that the number of veterans qualified for admission to the Hospital exceeded this figure and he further discovered that he had overlooked the gentlemen of the Life Guards and the yeomen of Horse in his calculations.

There had grown up since feudal times a rigid caste system in the army, symbolized by the right to possess and the ability to ride a horse. Thus the Life Guards were recruited from men 'of the best degree, for the meanest in one of these Troops is ever by his place a Gentleman, and so esteemed'. Many Life Guardsmen had in fact held commissions, and enjoyed a higher rate of pay than junior officers of Foot. Similarly, regiments of Horse were recruited from 'the best yeomen or best serving-men'. Dragoons, on the other hand, ranked not with the Horse, but with the Foot, for they were, in effect, mounted infantry, although they were paid 1*d.* a day more than foot-soldiers.

In fact, it was a fortunate oversight on Fox's part, for Life Guardsmen and troopers of Horse would never have condescended to share accommodation with common foot-soldiers, nor indeed to take meals with them. This Sir Christopher Wren now proceeded to remedy.

From each of the four pavilions at the ends of the two great wings, he projected an identical two-storey block, thus forming two new courts open respectively on their east and west sides. It was one of his happiest inspirations, for by so doing he increased the frontage of the Hospital and softened the severity of line of the main building. The result is both elegant and functional, for it solved the immediate problem of accommodation and at the same time caused Wren radically and impressively to alter the lay-out of his formal gardens. The south-east wing thus formed provided 'exclusive' wards for thirty-two Light Horsemen, while twenty-six 'officers', or Gentlemen of the Life Guards, were provided with quarters in the main pavilions. These grades require a brief explanation.

The twenty-six 'officers' were, in fact, non-commissioned officers

Light Horse Court. On the right the North-East wing, twice destroyed by enemy action of the Life Guards who for purposes of discipline were rated, and styled, as 'captains'. Light Horsemen were ex-cavalrymen who were admitted at a special rate of 2*s*. a week and whose persistent snobbery was to be the source of much head-breaking over the years. Both grades were abolished in 1850, some years after Lord John Russell's reforms. Within the original Hospital organization, three 'captains' were in charge of each of the eight companies of In-Pensioners, while the remaining two 'captains' were in nominal charge of the Light Horsemen.

Facing the Light Horse wards, from which the Court takes its name, were quarters for senior military and civilian staff. The other new quadrangle was later to be known as Infirmary Court for here, in the south-west block, Wren built an infirmary fitted up with thirty-two beds and with accommodation for the matron and nurses. This effectively replaced the unsatisfactory arrangement for the treatment of sick and infirm pensioners on the second floor of the north-east pavilion. Finally in the new north-west wing, Wren provided quarters for some of the under-officers and servants, and three dining-halls for the overflow of those who could not be accommodated in the Great Hall. These included the haughty cavalrymen who were provided with their own handsome 'Officers' Hall'.

With the building of a new Infirmary block in 1961 on the far side of the East Road, Infirmary Court was renamed College Court after the old Chelsea College which had stood upon this site three centuries before.

On July 5, 1686, James, during the course of a visit to his army encamped at Hounslow, studied and approved Wren's new proposals, and the following day he instructed Lord Ranelagh to make any payments as required 'for erecting such other buildings thereunto as we shall judge necessary'.

We must now return to the summer of 1685. The slow progress at Chelsea and the increasing number of old and infirm soldiers awaiting admission had begun to cause considerable hardship and discontent. James therefore moved fast. On July 21, only sixteen days after the battle of Sedgemoor, he issued a Royal Warrant setting out 'the Establishment and Regulation of Rewards and other Provisions to be made for His Majesties Land Forces', to take effect from the previous January 1 and to continue in the first instance until the opening of the Royal Hospital. Thus the system of Army pensions received its first formal blessing and whatever the blunders and shortcomings of James II, he should be remembered with gratitude for that sovereign act.

The Royal Warrant fell into three parts, dealing with 'Commission Officers wounded in fight', 'Non-commission Officers and Soldiers' and 'Rewards for Widdows, Orphans and Parents of such as are or shall be killed in His Majesty's Service'. We need concern ourselves only with the second category. Here the Warrant laid down that all non-commissioned officers and soldiers disabled by wounds or accidents should receive the following daily allowances *out of the funds appointed for the use of the hospital*:

A private soldier	5*d*.
A drummer	7*d*.
A sergeant	11*d*.
A corporal	7*d*.
One of the troops of the Guard	18*d*.
One of the Light Horse	12*d*.
A corporal of Light Horse	18*d*.
A dragoon	6*d*.
A corporal of dragoons	9*d*.
A master gunner	14*d*.
Another gunner	7*d*.

This provision was also extended to non-commissioned officers and soldiers who had served the Crown for twenty years, and who should come from any cause to be unfit for service. Finally, provision was made for a grant of 10*s*. towards a military funeral and this was claimed on behalf of 253 men who died during the following seven years, until the Hospital Burial Ground was taken into use.

The differential rates of pension set forth in the above table are a revealing indication of the 'class' structure of the early Regular Army (not, one might add, entirely eradicated in our own day and age). Predictably, the infantry private is at the bottom of the heap and, as we have seen, the gentleman of the Life Guards is at the top. In between are some nicely graded distinctions which must then have caused, as indeed they would today, a few regimental heart-burnings. But the rates, taken overall, were remarkably generous when it is remembered that as late as 1914, a private soldier's pay (before stoppages) was only 1*s.* a day, and his basic rate of service pension 6*d.* a day.

At the end of February, 1688, Lord Ranelagh reported to the King that 522 non-commissioned officers and men were then chargeable on the funds of the hospital at a cost of £5,002 0*s.* 5*d.* a year, besides 104 more described as 'entered for vacancies'. A year after the accession of William III, Lord Ranelagh reported again that there were then 579 pensioners and that since only 476 could be accommodated within the Royal Hospital, now approaching completion, 103 must continue to receive 'His Majesty's bounty in their quarters'. Hence the distinction between those pensioners who could be maintained within the Hospital and those who must remain outside, and so from December 10, 1689 the latter are described for the first time as *Out-Pensioners*.

Why the out-pension cost should have been made a charge on the Royal Hospital is not immediately apparent. So long as the numbers remained small, there was no great strain upon Hospital funds. But after Marlborough's wars, and despite the fact that, with the formation of the Royal Regiment of Artillery and the conversion of engineers from a civilian to a military corps, the Out-Pensioners of both were transferred to the Board of Ordnance, the total of other Out-Pensioners began to reach proportions far beyond the financial or administrative resources of the Chelsea Board, as the following brief table shows:

Out-Pensioners

1692		98
1702		51
1773		16,007
1873		66,281
1973	(approx.)	228,000

The derisory figures up to 1702 are an indication of the deliberate and mischievous practices of Lord Ranelagh; the 1773 figure shows the effect of thirty years of military involvement overseas; in 1847, some years after the administration of Kilmainham Out-Pensioners had been transferred to the Chelsea Board, the cost of the Royal Hospital and all its pension responsibilities was met entirely out of Parliamentary Votes and so the 1873 figure is merely a numerical reflection of a more liberal policy and of Victoria's colonial wars; finally in 1955, all responsibility for out-pensions was transferred to two Government departments – service pensions to the Army Pensions Office and disability pensions to the Department of Health and Social Security. The total figure for 1973 shown above (which includes both service and disability pensioners) is a reasonably accurate approximation and serves to underline the massive impact of two world wars.

By the end of 1685, the extension of the Royal Hospital was being planned and the pension scheme had been set in train. Through his son, Charles, who was still Paymaster-General, Sir Stephen Fox was able effectively to control the progress of events at Chelsea; but in November, unable to reconcile his conscience with the King's proposed expansion of the standing army, Charles Fox was 'put out of the Pay Office'. In his place – and at the suggestion of Lawrence Hyde, now Earl of Rochester – James appointed Lord Ranelagh. It was to prove a disastrous choice.

Richard Jones, first and only Earl of Ranelagh, came of a prominent Irish family. His father, the second Viscount, had already shown a flexible talent for hunting with Cromwell and running with the Royalists, and the son soon proved himself no less adept. At the age of twenty-eight the Duke of Ormonde appointed him Chancellor of the Irish Exchequer. It was Ranelagh's first involvement with public money and it provided him with an appetite which grew with the lushness of each succeeding pasture. When, thirty-four years later, he was dismissed from the Pay Office and expelled from Parliament, his army accounts were in arrears to the tune of over £5,000,000, and revealed a cool misappropriation of £72,000. Yet this irrepressible rogue, only a few months later, was made a Governor of Queen Anne's Bounty, 'for the augmentation of the maintenance of poor clergy' and in 1708 was reappointed to the Privy Council. To the end he remained impenitent. Here he is in 1711, eight months before his death, writing to Lowndes, Secretary of the Treasury:

'My necessities are so great and pressing that I must desyre you as my old and true friend to move my Lord Treasurer even this morning, to order mee a supply for myself and clerks. I wayted upon his Lordsp this very morning, and hee was pleased to give mee what I thought was some assurance of his goodness to mee. But you know that fayre words will neither pay clerkes nor goe to markett, and that while the grasse is growing the horse may

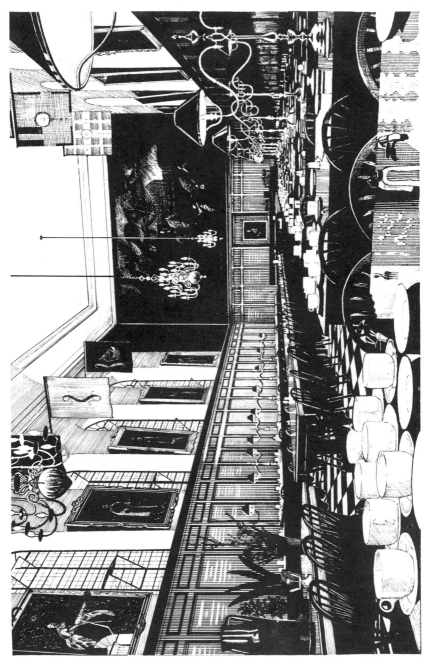

The Great Hall

starve. This is really and truly my case, for I have neither place nor pension, with seaventy yeares and a great many debts upon my back and nothing to trust to but a small Irish estate ill payd. Pray therefore, my dear Lowndes, bee a speedy and earnest sollicitor for your poor old and true servant

Ranelagh'

In this instance 'fayre words' went to market with a vengeance, for they extracted for Lord Ranelagh upwards of £5,000 from the Treasury. The best that can be said of this outrageous man is that, in an age of villainy, he was a whale among minnows.

Ranelagh's technique was simple and consisted of establishing himself in the favour of the person who mattered most, the King. The fact that he won the confidence and support of three men so totally different as Charles II, James II and William III is a tribute as much to his versatility as to his Irish blarney. Thus after a visit to London in 1670, he persuaded Charles to appoint him Vice-Treasurer of Ireland, in which capacity he behaved with the utmost irregularity, contrived to bring about the dismissal of Ormonde, and impudently offered to provide Charles with the money to rebuild Windsor Castle out of the Irish revenue. Eventually, with the law breathing down his neck, he took refuge in London whither in 1680 he was pursued by an action for the fraudulent conversion of £76,000. This left him undismayed, for in the meantime he had purchased from the Earl of Sunderland a cosy billet at Court as Gentleman of the Bedchamber and from this strategic position, and with the help of Lawrence Hyde, he secured from the King a suspension of the action *and* – with typical effrontery – an annuity of £300 out of the Irish revenue! Such was the man to whose tender mercies the Royal Hospital was now committed.

To begin with, Ranelagh moved with circumspection. His time was largely occupied with the financial administration of James's expanding army and he was shrewd enough not to reveal his hand to Wren or to Stephen Fox. Nonetheless, he introduced a crony of his, Ralph Cooke, to oversee his interests at the Royal Hospital. This distasteful character, cast in his master's mould, progressed by way of the Stewardship to the office of Deputy Treasurer, in which capacity he successfully lined his own pocket until in 1702 the same chopper which cut short the Paymaster's activities also put an end to his own.

Ranelagh's salary at the Pay Office was £2,000 (equivalent to £30,000 a year tax-free today), but he considered that no more than pin-money. He was playing for much higher stakes and after his fall, John Macky observed: '. . . (he) hath spent more money, built more fine houses and laid out more on household furniture than any other nobleman in England. He is a great epicure and prodigious expensive.'

It was not until 1688 that Ranelagh turned his full attention to Chelsea. Some time during that year, despite the fact that he already had a palatial residence in Whitehall and had appropriated the Steward's apartments at Chelsea, Wren designed for him an elegant house with extensive outbuildings in the Hospital grounds opposite the east end of the Light Horse wards. We do not know on what authority Wren put this work in hand, but he was an ingenuous and honest man and we may be sure that Ranelagh manufactured a persuasive and watertight case. At his examination in 1702, he claimed repeatedly that the house, its gardens, its sumptuous furnishings and its magnificent collection of paintings had been provided entirely out of his own pocket. But in the Hospital accounts for 1688–9 there is a discrepancy of £10,322 4s. 4d. and a reference to 'diverse other works' and there can be no doubt that Ranelagh House was built out of Hospital funds. Not even this wily operator would have spent his own money erecting a house on land which he did not own and to which he could as yet claim no title.

Ranelagh's preoccupation with his Chelsea house was also one of the main reasons for the delay in admitting the first In-Pensioners to the Hospital. The sixteen original wards were all ready for occupation by the end of 1689, but to have gone ahead at that time would have interfered with the improvements and embellishments to his own property. It would also have diverted far too much of the available money to its proper object. Thus – and it was by no means for the last time – the pensioners were made to suffer for the Paymaster's private greed and corruption.

During this same year, Ranelagh set forth in a long memorandum to the King his proposals for reducing the number of men for whom immediate accommodation was not available in the Hospital. His recommendations seemed innocent enough, but where money was concerned, Ranelagh was never innocent. His object was more devious, for by reducing the out-pension charge on Hospital funds to its lowest possible level, he could retain a greater sum for his own nefarious purposes.

As the year ran its course, James began to encounter serious political difficulties at home and abroad, a situation of which Ranelagh was quick to take advantage. In July, he brazenly appropriated the sum of £6,322, which represented the balance of the poundage fund attributable to the Royal Hospital for the years 1686–7, on the extremely flimsy pretext of his costs incurred when encamped with the army at Hounslow and 'the constant trouble and attendance I underwent in looking after the Concernes of the Royall Hospitall near Chelsea, for which I had no manner of advantage.'

In November, he went one better. Shortly after William of Orange landed at Torbay, James moved his headquarters to Salisbury and his Paymaster dutifully followed him there with a large retinue of clerks. Four months later he petitioned King William to allow him to keep the 1688 balance of Exchequer fees amounting to £6,911 'in view of the very great Expense for my Equipage to Salisbury'. As Dean remarks, it must have been the biggest claim in history for a week's travelling expenses. And riding his luck, this egregious rascal at the same time asked that his salary should be increased to £3,000 to bring him in line with the Treasurer of the Navy 'who had not halfe so much Buisnesse.' Nor, one might add, half so much nerve. The King agreed to both these requests without question, partly because he did not yet know Ranelagh's reputation and partly because he was preoccupied with other matters. He had also dismissed from the Treasury a month earlier Sir Stephen Fox, the one man who might have told him the truth.

Ranelagh now turned his attention to an even more ambitious idea. He had a house at Chelsea, but no security of tenure. Accordingly in February, 1690 he submitted a petition for a long lease of 7 acres of land lying to the south of Light Horse Court on part of which he had already built his house and which included an essential element of Wren's formal garden plan. Two months later he was granted a sixty-one year lease at £15 7s. 6d. a year, despite the fact that this was twice the term of Crown leases permitted by Act of Parliament. There is clear evidence here of collusion with William Jephson, the Secretary of the Treasury, who one month later obtained an identical lease on the western side of the Royal Hospital.

But the insatiable Earl had not finished yet. In May, 1696 he petitioned for the *freehold* of a further 15 acres lying to the south-east of the Hospital and eventually was granted a ninety-nine-year lease for the princely sum of £5 per annum. He returned to the charge

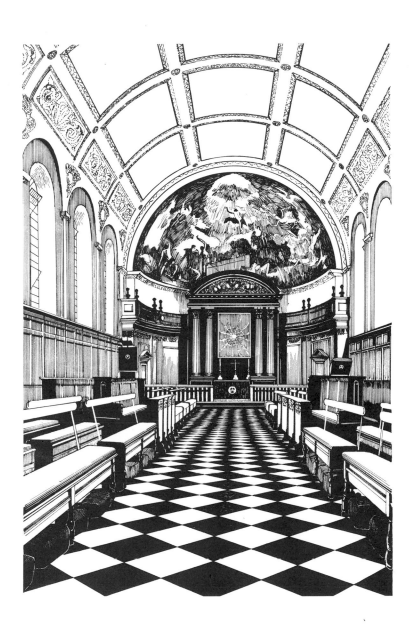

The Chapel

again the following April, supporting his claim 'as being compensation for losses sustained to my property by the late war in Ireland'. This time his persistence and his glib tongue were rewarded, for he obtained a grant in fee in perpetuity of both leaseholds in consideration of an annual rent to the Royal Hospital of £5 a year! Thus, without a blow being struck, the Hospital surrendered nearly one-third of its entire property. In due course, between the years 1742 and 1857, the Commissioners re-acquired virtually the whole Ranelagh estate by purchase. It cost them £35,317 6s. 7d. – which would have greatly amused the first Earl of Ranelagh.

There we will leave him for the moment. We shall meet him again, sharp and devious as ever, in the next chapter when the Royal Hospital is opened and the pensioners have taken the centre of the stage.

Fortunately not all of James II's appointments at Chelsea were out of the same mould as the wicked Earl. Of these, five are of particular interest.

Matthew Ingram had been commissioned into the Coldstream Guards and in June, 1685 was appointed Captain and Adjutant to the Colonel of his Regiment, the Earl of Craven, at that time acting as the equivalent of G.O.C., London District. With the introduction of the new pension scheme in the summer of 1685, it became necessary to find an officer to act as the pensioners' paymaster and to supervise them in their quarters until such time as the Hospital was ready to receive them. Ingram was clearly nominated for these duties by Craven who, for all his 75 years, was a lively old soldier and highly regarded by the King. He had also been a modest contributor to the original Hospital subscription fund.

It was an admirable choice, and for Ingram it started a nine-year association with Chelsea. Not only were the pensioners regularly and properly paid (a situation which was not destined to last for long) but the worthy Ingram, with a Guardsman's eye for regimental efficiency, immediately arranged to have his ragged flock re-clothed and their hair cut. The old soldiers were still dressed in what remained of their old and various regimentals and by a happy inspiration Ingram persuaded the King to allow them to wear the scarlet and blue previously granted only to Royal regiments. Thus the In-Pensioners today owe to James II the privilege of wearing the royal livery. No visual record of the Ingram uniforms has survived, but we may assume that they provided the model for the three versions of In-Pensioners' dress laid down in 1692.

In 1690, Matthew Ingram was appointed to fill the position of Major at the Royal Hospital and three months before the In-Pensioners took up residence he was chosen to be the first Major and Lieutenant-Governor. Among many acts of benefaction, he presented the first organ for the chapel and when he died in 1694, the Hospital lost a devoted and distinguished servant.

The King now turned his attention to the appointment of a Governor. He had before him the administrative model of the Invalides and also of Kilmainham Hospital, where a Master had been appointed a year before the building was opened. The qualifications for the Kilmainham post required that the selected officer should be, among other things, 'a Protestant, a gentleman, over fifty years of age . . . and unmarried'. So far as is known, no such specifics were laid down for Chelsea and it is certainly most unlikely that James would have insisted on a *Protestant* Governor there, at the very time when he was busy appointing Catholics to high public office.

There does not seem to have been any stampede to obtain the appointment, for the salary of £300 a year was the same as that of an infantry Colonel though without the 'fringe benefits' available to the latter. It was not until some years afterwards that the full possibilities of the Governorship at Chelsea as a source of rich perquisites became apparent.

The first officer to be selected was Sir Thomas Daniell who had been knighted for distinguished services as a cavalry Colonel in the Civil War. Thereafter he had held a series of minor commands in backwater garrisons and appears to have been a safe but uninspired choice. At the time of his appointment he was aged 72. He had also not been paid for two years, a fact which he was attempting to rectify through the good offices of Sir Stephen Fox, when in October he suddenly died.

He was replaced by Sir Thomas Ogle who had spent most of the Civil War in captivity or as one of the exiled King's intelligence agents in London. He had subsequently fallen out of favour with Charles after a drunken orgy in Bow Street during which he and his companions had exposed themselves indecently on the tavern balcony, to the delight of the crowd and the indignation of the authorities. Though disgraced, he obtained a commission in the 3rd Foot (the Buffs), only for his company to mutiny while preparing to embark for Ostend. Thus in the autumn of 1685, by which time he

93

A Village in Chelsea

had arrived painfully at the rank of Lt. Colonel, it could hardly be
said that his military service had been particularly distinguished. On
his appointment to Chelsea, he surrendered his commission, for
which unusually selfless act he was rewarded with a pension of £200
in addition to his salary. He seems to have made little mark on
the Royal Hospital and he must have been fortunate to have had
as his deputy an officer of such outstanding qualities as Matthew
Ingram.

The three remaining 'foundation members' were all related,
though they curiously chose to spell their names differently.

The first of these was Dr Charles Fraiser who was appointed
Physician in May, 1687. His father had been personal physician to
Charles II in exile and he himself became one of the King's medical
advisers after the Restoration and also something rather more than
medical adviser to two of the royal mistresses. He was clearly a man
of ability, for his court appointment was confirmed by James II and
on the accession of King William, he was promoted to Second
Physician, which post he combined with his Royal Hospital duties
until the autumn of 1693 when he appears to have lost his reason and
was replaced by the celebrated Theodore Colladon.

In November, 1687, the Rev. Augustine Frezer was appointed
Chaplain. Thus, in keeping with the origin and purpose of the
Hospital, both the physical and spiritual welfare of the In-Pensioners
were catered for at the outset. Augustine Frezer probably owed his
appointment to the recommendation of his cousin, Charles, and
since the consecration of the Chapel took place in August, 1691, he
could be said to have been the first officiating member of the Royal
Hospital staff. As we shall see in the next chapter, his duties as laid
down in the Hospital Instruction Book of 1692 kept both him and
his 'curat' fully occupied. Perhaps too occupied, for in 1699 he
resigned his chaplaincy for a less onerous cure of souls in Essex. Of
all the vanished images of the early days of Chelsea, that of divine
service under Augustine Frezer would be worth recapturing.
Chapel attendance was compulsory (as it is today), though one
imagines it was a rule more honoured in the breach than the
observance; at the organ, Peter Dumas, the first to hold that
appointment; the old soldiers provided with prayer-books (at 13s.
each) which they could not read, and entertained with sermons
which they probably could not understand; while from the cellars
below came those sounds of merriment and tippling which later
caused the Commissioners to wax exceeding wrathful.

The third of the Frasers was James 'Catalogue' Fraser who was

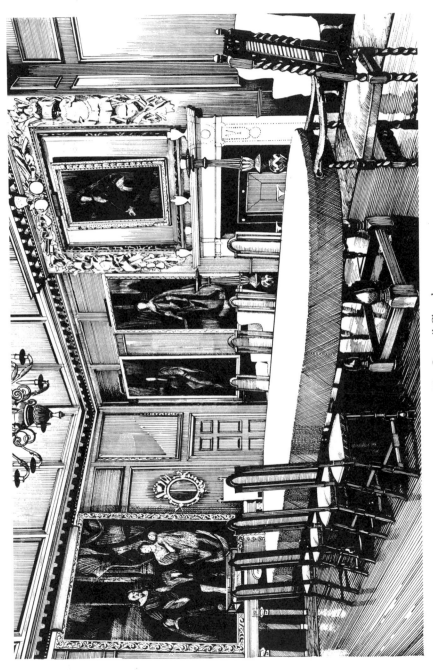

The Council Chamber

appointed Secretary and Register in September, 1688 'in consideration of a Debt due to him from the Crown'. This was probably a reference to his services in managing, at some cost to himself, Nell Gwyn's financial affairs after the death of Charles II. He was by trade an antiquarian bookseller and as remote from the world of old soldiers as any man could be. He occupied an apartment at the Royal Hospital for thirty years, during the first half of which his duties were performed by his clerk, and thereafter by three successive deputies. He was very much a product of his times and we shall meet him again.

Thus, as we reach the end of the year 1688, the stage is nearly set and the chief actors are about to take their places. Yet before the curtain could rise, the impresario had fled the scene. On December 4, at the second attempt, James II succeeded in making his ignominious escape to join his wife and the infant prince and future Old Pretender in Paris. Once more the Royal Hospital found itself under new management.

6

'Perfecere Gulielmus et Maria, Rex et Regina'

❦

The man who succeeded James II was a strange, sombre figure.
William of Orange was small, pock-marked, asthmatic and racked by
a persistent cough. From early manhood he had known only the
grim face of war and the devious patterns of domestic and European
politics; now, in middle life, he had become solitary and ruthless,
loveless and largely unloved. He was the complete antithesis of
Charles II and the one quality he had in common with James was a
total lack of humour. It is difficult to think of any man more ill-
suited to rule the English.

His claim to the throne was tenuous by any hereditary law, but
the English genius for compromise contrived the idea of joint
sovereignty with his wife Mary and thus secured the Protestant
succession through her sister Anne in spite of every effort by the
Jacobite faction to restore the crown to James and his heirs. William
disliked England and detested the English people. But throughout
his life he was driven by a burning sense of mission to destroy French
domination of Europe; and to do this, he needed the English fleet
and the support of English arms. To this end, he was prepared to
swallow his pride and his distaste for all things English. He was a
brave, but not a great commander; he was a shrewd but not a
brilliant political tactician; and though a sternly Calvinist Protestant,
he had no religious prejudice towards Catholicism other than the
fact that it was the religion of his sworn enemy, Louis XIV. For
over half his reign he was involved in war with France and under
his leadership a raw and largely untrained army received its first
bitter baptism of fire in Flanders – that bloodstained battleground
to which it was to return many times in the years ahead and where it
was to win an indelible renown. The Treaty of Ryswick in 1697
brought an uneasy peace; but before the final confrontation with
France, William was dead. The torch he had carried with such
singleness of purpose for thirty years now passed to the greatest of
all English military commanders.

❦

Once again the Royal Hospital was fortunate, for William – like James II – was a soldier-King. At his examination in 1702, Lord Ranelagh recorded that 'King William, upon his coming to the Crown, visited the said Hospital and renewed the former directions for the speedy finishing and furnishing of it'. A month after his accession William had indeed visited Chelsea and had expressed his approval of the buildings, which now included Wren's first extensions, and two of the original wards which Ranelagh had craftily furnished and equipped, if only to disarm any criticism that he was dragging his feet. The King's directions for 'the speedy finishing and furnishing' of the Hospital cut very little ice with Ranelagh. He had twice ignored similar instructions from James and now events conspired in his favour. The dismissal of Stephen Fox in February left him virtually a free hand; and with the outbreak of war with France in May, the King had other and more pressing matters on his mind. So for another twelve months Ranelagh occupied himself happily with the development of his Chelsea property and the unfortunate pensioners languished in their quarters while their village slumbered.

Meanwhile Wren pressed forward with the completion of the buildings and the laying out of the gardens. By now the Hospital itself was finished so far as the accommodation and entertainment of the pensioners was concerned. But a village needs its communal services and these Wren now provided. On the far side of the West Road, beyond College Court, he added a whole range of administrative buildings. We need not concern ourselves here with their every detail, for a century later they were to be almost totally destroyed by Sir John Soane in an access of misplaced architectural zeal; but they included a magnificent stable-yard, a washhouse and drying yard, two guardhouses, a coal yard, a bakery and – since Wren had learned a thing or two about old soldiers – a brewery. In addition, he built an 'Elabritory' on the east side in which the Apothecary could distil his various potions, and a number of small dwellings for members of the Hospital staff. But predictably he encountered a stumbling-block.

In order to complete his plans for this new development, he had persuaded Stephen Fox some years earlier to purchase from Lord Cheyne a plot of four and a half acres known as Great Swede Court on the western side of the Hospital. This would have given him the room he needed in which to spread himself, but he had not reckoned with Lord Ranelagh and his friends. As we have seen, shortly after Ranelagh had obtained his first lease on the opposite side of the

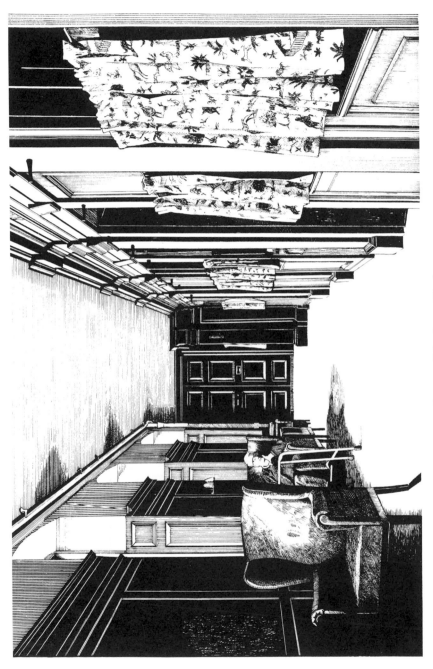

In one of the Long Wards

Hospital property, his partner in crime, William Jephson, acquired the tenancy of Great Swede Court at the nominal rent of £9 a year. Jephson was on safe ground. Not only had he been secretary to William of Orange before the Revolution, but he was now Secretary of the Treasury and keeper of the Secret Service Fund. He was thus virtually in the position of holding a blank cheque signed by the King. What happened to Wren's precious acres is another story – and for that we must await the entry in due course of Sir Robert Walpole.

In spite of Jephson, Wren had virtually completed the final extensions by the end of 1691. And simultaneously he had been working on his grand design for the grounds and gardens, a setting worthy of his splendid buildings and destined to be largely ruined by Victorian vandals and modern urban development.

To create a proper sense of space on the north side, Wren matched the widened frontage of the Hospital with 'a great Court enclosed before it'. This was Burton's Court, purchased from Lord Cheyne in 1687, and here Wren built two lodges and imposing entrance gates. To conform to his plan, the highway from Chelsea to Westminster was closed and a new road constructed round the Court. This main entrance was approached by a broad avenue which led to the King's Private Road and may well have been intended as the first stage of a royal carriageway leading to William III's palace of Kensington. Burton's Court was laid out 'with beautiful walks and plantacons' and with avenues of trees so placed that they did not obscure the vista of the north front and its imposing portico, an effect now destroyed by the central avenue of limes planted in 1888 with a fine Victorian disregard for taste or perspective.

Wren had given his Royal Hospital a royal approach. Now he gave it a royal outlook to the river. Beyond Figure Court he designed an ornamental water garden. Along the south front a wide terrace descended to a water gate on the river, flanked by two charming summerhouses. The water gate (which served as a southern entrance to the Hospital for river-borne visitors) was approached by a raised causeway running between two 40-foot wide canals (later extended along the south terrace) on either side of which were plantations of fruit and flowering trees lined by herbaceous borders. The effect was to give an English informality to a formal French design. Beyond this elegant and charming garden, on the east and west sides, Wren enclosed, between brick walls and quickset hedges, the Apothecary's 'physic garden' and plots for the supply of vegetables for the Great Kitchen and potherbs for those pensioners who preferred a more innocent brew than strong ale. The village setting was complete.*

Wren laid great store by his formal gardens. Work was begun in 1687 and took five years, in spite, or perhaps because, of Lord Ranelagh's intrusions with his own property development, and although no exact accounts have survived, the cost must have been at least £20,000. Little of his grand design remains today, but that, too – as we shall see – is another story.

The reappointment of Stephen Fox as a Treasury Commissioner in February, 1690 must have been unwelcome news for Lord Ranelagh who had good reason to fear the return of the Hospital's old watchdog. Fox wasted little time, for the following month the King directed Ranelagh to give a full account – in writing – of his stewardship. The Paymaster duly presented a long, tendentious report the main burden of which was a request for an additional allocation of poundage in the sum of £10,374 to meet the Hospital budget. That this sum almost exactly represented the cost of building Ranelagh House is something more than a coincidence.

Ranelagh further reported that the pension list numbered 579 old soldiers of whom only 474 could be accommodated in the Hospital (with characteristically shaky arithmetic he wrongly cast up the total as 472!) and suggested that the remaining 105 Out-Pensioners might sensibly be re-examined with a view to their being discharged 'as being yet well able to serve your Majestie either at sea or in the garrisons'.

Finally, he aimed a couple of poisoned darts at his predecessor, Charles Fox, and at Christopher Wren, both designed to underline his own impeccable honesty and his selfless devotion to duty. His claim to have been 'the sole mover and diligent overseer of the building and finishing of ye Royal Hospital' stung the mild-mannered Wren to action.

Neither at Chelsea, nor later at Greenwich, was Wren paid a penny for his services as architect and supervisor, considering them both to be charitable institutions for which he was privileged to give his time and talents without reward. But he had his professional

* See p. 64.

pride and six months after the Hospital was opened he petitioned the
Privy Council 'to order such allowance as your Commissioners of
the Treasury shall think reasonable for my Expence in 10 years
attendance on so considerable a building'. A year went by before the
Treasury agreed that he should be awarded £1,000 'for his great
Care and Paines in Directing and Overseeing the Building of the
said Hospitall'. It was something of a back-handed compliment, for
the Treasury directed that the fee should be paid out of the Hospital's overstretched funds.

Ranelagh must have laughed loudly at this. Not for him petitions
to the Privy Council. Four years earlier, as we have seen, he had
simply appropriated over £6,000 of the poundage fund as compensation for his own alleged 'Diligence in Directing and Overseeing the Building of the said Hospitall'.

The Paymaster's report to the King was duly pigeon-holed
(probably to Ranelagh's relief) but the matter of the pensioners
surplus to the Chelsea establishment was dealt with – albeit many
months later – by the formation of a Company of Invalids to carry
out guard duties at Windsor Castle. The history of Invalid Companies lies outside the scope of this book, but we may note here that
they were an ingenious device for providing inexpensive garrisons
at key points throughout the country and for reducing the charge for
out-pensions when money was short. Their number fluctuated
throughout the next century until their final disbandment in 1803;
for example, the 41st Foot (Invalids) and twenty-five independent
companies were raised in 1721, and five more companies in 1740;
fourteen were disbanded in 1764 after the Seven Years War; and
twelve were re-formed in 1794. Their military capability must have
been severely limited and their conduct reprehensible, for an eye-
witness reported in 1723 that the garrison of Upnor Castle on the
Medway consisted of 'men so decay'd and decrepit that they are
scarcely able to move body and soul together to those disreputable
taverns which they so riotously frequent'. Their memory is still
celebrated today on the uniform buttons worn by In-Pensioners
which bear the letters R.C.I. (Royal Company of Invalids) surmounted by a crown.

The shelving of Ranelagh's report left the Hospital in the state of
suspended animation which had existed since the last months of
James II's reign. On April 27, 1691, during a brief visit to England,
William 'dined at Lord Ranelagh's at Chelsea Colledge'. Ranelagh
took this opportunity to solicit the King's agreement to his being
paid £1 a day for his services as Treasurer of the Hospital, back-

dated to December, *1685*. The opening of the Hospital was not discussed.

By the summer of 1691, Stephen Fox's patience must have been exhausted. Although the King was still abroad, Fox enlisted the support of the Secretary of State, the Earl of Nottingham, and together they prevailed upon Queen Mary to issue a series of Royal Warrants, designed to put an end to Lord Ranelagh's delaying tactics. Two of these Warrants allocated two-thirds of the poundage fund to the Hospital, back-dated to January, 1688, and this produced £60,825, enough to pay off the arrears due to the building contractors.

The third Warrant, dated August 12, directed the Bishop of London to proceed with the consecration of the chapel and the burial ground. As we have seen, the service of consecration took place on August 30 and was followed by 'an entertainment', for providing which Roger Hewitt, the future Clerk of the Works, was paid £19 1s. 6d. It must have been a monumental feast.

Finally – and most significantly – a fourth Warrant was issued on August 14, appointing as acting Commissioners Lord Ranelagh, Sir Stephen Fox and Sir Christopher Wren and directing them to take all necessary steps to bring the Hospital into use. The Warrant was very specific and bears all the hallmarks of Fox's attention to detail. The Commissioners were required, among other things, to arrange for 'the dyet of such persons as are to be entertained and fed in Our said Royall Hospitall, and to make contracts . . . for furnishing the same . . . as also for cloathing the said persons, and washing the linen, and keeping in good order the severall courts, gardens, walks and avenues . . .' They were further to produce accounts of all expenditure on building and furnishing to the end of 1690 and of all wages and salaries paid, or due, to existing staff. Finally, they were to draw up an establishment for In-Pensioners and staff with proposed rates of pay, fill any outstanding vacancies, and draft a set of 'house instructions'.

Fox and Wren acted without delay and within a month had entered into contracts with George London and Henry Wise for the upkeep of the gardens, and with the Whitster for laundry services. The latter was a fixed rate contract and the Whitster, who was paid a small allowance and provided with furnished rooms, was kept remarkably busy, for in the June quarter of 1696, he washed no fewer than 37,436 articles. Cleanliness at Chelsea seems to have taken precedence even over godliness.

On September 18, the catering arrangements were made and the wording of each contract specified the closest possible attention to quality. As we have noted earlier, both Fox and Wren were obviously determined that the old soldiers should be entertained in a manner befitting a royal establishment. The butcher's contract for 'beefe, mutton and veale' was worth £1,369 for the year, which represented 1s. a week for each In-Pensioner and member of the staff. Since beef and mutton cost 3d. a pound, it can be seen that no one was likely to starve. The cheesemonger's contract called for salt butter to be supplied at 5d. a pound and best Gloucestershire cheese at 3d., while the fishmonger's Friday offering of salted fish was costed at 2½d. a pound.* Finally the contract for bread and beer was given to one, John England, who rather unwisely was then appointed Master Butler and Baker to the Hospital.

While Fox and Wren were thus occupied, Ranelagh watched from the sidelines. He alone was in a position to produce the accounts as directed under the Warrant and not for the first – and certainly not for the last – time he entirely ignored his instructions. He turned his attention instead to the furnishing of the buildings. This was clearly Wren's responsibility, but for Ranelagh it presented too good an opportunity to miss and he poached on the architect's territory with relish. Apart from extracting a commission out of the various contractors, he succeeded in channelling over half the goods supplied into Ranelagh House and thus his own cut of the total bill of £5,899 was of the order of £3,000 in cash and kind. Since the accounts were not passed for seven years, Wren could only guess at the extent of his colleague's malpractices.

Thus by the end of the year the village was virtually ready to receive its In-Pensioners. On January 1, 1692 the King approved the Hospital establishment. This is set out in detail on p. 105, together with the comparative establishment as authorized exactly one hundred years later.

The 1692 establishment was experimental. The remarkable fact is that it changed so little in the next hundred years – a net increase of only six people. The salary scales, however, are more revealing. Despite the fact that by 1792 the pound was worth only 13s. com-

---

* For some unexplained reason, fish disappeared from the In-Pensioners' diet in 1747 and was not resumed until the present century.

COMPARATIVE ESTABLISHMENT, ROYAL HOSPITAL

	1692 £ s. d.	1792 £ s. d.	
Governor as Governor ⎫	300		
more as pension ⎬	200	500	
Lieut. Governor ⎫		200	
Major ⎭	100	100	
Chaplain	100	100	
Curat (Second Chaplain)	80	100	
Phisitian	100	100	
Secretary ⎫	80	100	
Clerk ⎭	20	—	
Deputy Treasurer	80	100	
Steward	50	100	
Comptroller	40	100	
Clerk of the Works	20	20	
Chirurgeon	73	100	
Apothecary	50	50	
Adjutant	—	60	
Men Servants (all with dyett)			
Deputy Clerk of the Works	13 6 8	—	
Chirurgeon's Mate	20	20	
Wardrobe Keeper ⎫		20	
Comptroller of Coal Yard ⎭	40	30	
Master Cooke	40	40	
Second Master Cooke	30	30	
Sculleryman	20	20	
Three under cookes at £10	30	30	
Master Butler ⎫		40	and one servant
⎬	40		
Master Baker ⎭		50	and three servants (one only)
Three under butlers at £10	30	25	
Three under bakers at £10	30	—	
Sexton	16	20	
Usher of the Hall	12	20	
Yeoman of the coal yard	20	—	
Porter	12	12	
Two sweepers at £10	20	20	
Lamplighter	—	20	
Chirurgeon's Deputy	—	20	
Two under scullerymen at £10	—	20	
Gardener	—	20	
Messenger	—	20	
Organist	—	20	
Women Servants (all with dyett)			
Housekeeper	30	30	
Underhousekeeper	20	—	
24 Matrons at £8	192	192	
	Without dyett	*With dyett*	
Barber and servants	60	60	
Cannall keeper and turncock	20	20	
	£1,988 6 8	£2,529 0 0	

pared with a century before, the majority of the servants were still being paid at the original rates, while the salaries of officers and senior staff throw up some odd anomalies, chiefly due to the patronage practices of the day.

In the first establishment it had been specifically laid down that the increment of £200 given to Sir Thomas Ogle by way of pension was for life 'but not to be continued to any succeeding Governor'. It was to prove a pious intention, for it was continued to his successor, Colonel Hales; to Colonel Hales's successor; and to *his* successor's successor; at which point the Treasury gave up the unequal struggle and consolidated the increment into the Governor's salary. Similarly, it was laid down that on the 'death or other determination' of the Secretary – the non-effective 'Catalogue' Fraser – the post would be abolished and the duties performed by the clerk. In the event, it was the clerk who was abolished.

It proved to be the last calm before the storm, for in the new establishment that followed William Windham's Act of 1806, the staff was increased to eighty-eight, and the salary bill jumped to £9,175 10*s*. It has never looked back.

On February 4, 1692, after what must have seemed to them an eternity, the first group of In-Pensioners was admitted to the Hospital. The nominal roll of these men has survived and shows that all of them, ninety-nine in number, were severely disabled by wounds, old age or other infirmities; and the fact that twenty-five of them were at once committed to the Infirmary suggests that they were the most urgent and deserving cases. An odd footnote to their arrival is the request a few days later to Charles Hopson, Deputy Clerk of the Works, to provide an assortment of 'Coffins, Crutches, Wooden Leggs and ashen Stumps, Feather Pillows, Leather Girdles and all sorts of trusses for Lame and Bursten men'. They were in every sense the halt, the lame and the blind.

Finally, on March 28, the remaining 377 In-Pensioners took up residence. It must have been a great day for Fox and Wren who had laboured so devotedly for ten long years to honour Charles II's pledge to his old soldiers. There is no record of any formal opening ceremony, for the King, as usual, was abroad and the process of moving in must have fully occupied both pensioners and staff.

The old men must have looked in wonder at their new surroundings for none of them could have experienced such comparative luxury before. Here, probably for the first time, they had a home of their own, comfortable beds, linen sheets, proper washing facilities, and attendants to wait upon them in their quarters. Even if their pay was only a few pence a week, at least they received it regularly – and in full. And they were under the humane and watchful eye of the kindly Matthew Ingram. Their one complaint was probably that it was a long walk to the nearest ale-house.

It was the same in the Great Hall. Here they messed by wards at sixteen long tables, with linen table-cloths and a fine pewter service. They were provided with spoons but no knives and forks, which suggests that they used the former to negotiate their gruel and burgooe, and for the rest resorted to their fingers. Over all – at least in the early days – was an air of monastic discipline, as witness the Instruction Book:

'1. That the Serjeants daily attend in the Hall at Dinner and Supper Time.

'2. That they constantly and gravely say Grace at the Head of their Tables.

'3. That they make the men at their Tables behave with Order, Silence and Decency.'

Food was served in strict rotation: first the unsociable cavalrymen in their Officers' Hall; then the other In-Pensioners in the Great Hall; next the Governor's table; and finally the House-keeper's and Servants' Halls. The daily ration scale was generous – 12 oz. of meat per man (Sergeants and above received an extra 4 oz.), fish on the same scale on Fridays, two loaves of bread, ¼ lb. of butter, ¼ lb. of cheese, two quarts of beer, and a liberal supply of vegetables. No meal was complete without quantities of mustard to camouflage the taste of stale or corrupt meat. This diet was excessive for old men unused to such extravagance and soon there grew up that traffic in surplus food which was to become a standard practice at the Hospital until quite recent times.* In the early days it was a firm market, for threepence-worth of meat translated into six quarts of beer – a fair exchange, even if there was a hint of robbery.

* R.S.M. Ives, a legendary figure at Chelsea, recalls that on his arrival at the Hospital in 1954, he noticed gaps in the hedge bordering on Royal Hospital Road. On inquiry, he discovered that these were the channels through which In-Pensioners' rations found their way to the citizenry outside.

William III's soldiers were a rough lot. From small beginnings, the standing army had grown until by 1694 there were 90,000 men under arms. The increase had far outstripped the ability of the administrative services to cope, with the result that corruption and inefficiency were the order of the day and the contractor system for clothing and rations provided some rich pickings. It is a wonder that the army was ever fit to go to war. It is an even greater wonder that it managed to fight when it got there.

In theory, this was a 'volunteer' army, but old soldiers will know the infinitely delicate shades of meaning which have attached themselves to that word. Recruiting methods were devious and distasteful for this was the period of the 'crimping' establishments through which men were decoyed into the service by a variety of subterfuges of which alcoholic remorse was the most conventional and the payment of a King's bounty the most effective. As a result, the ranks were filled from the most dissolute elements of society among which convicted felons were predominant. No questions were asked. No medical standards were required. It was in every sense a 'brutal and licentious soldiery'. This soldiery was distinguished by two characteristics which were to be the hallmarks of the British army for many years: a compulsive addiction to alcohol and a breathtaking obscenity of language. Indeed, a contemporary has described William III's expeditionary force in what must be the shortest and most succinct of all campaign reports: 'The Army went to Flanders and swore horribly.' This army was the terror of the Low Countries. No woman was safe. No property was sacrosanct. It was not the British army's finest hour.

Yet it was redeemed by one shining virtue which survived every tribulation. When battle was joined, this ill-trained, ill-disciplined and ill-led* army displayed a gallantry in action and a fortitude in adversity which were the envy of its allies and the wonder of its enemies. The Mutiny Act had legalized the position of the armed forces of the Crown. It had also laid down a savage code of punishment which reduced men to the status of animals and handed down a sentence of 300 lashes as a minimum corrective. That Marlborough, ten years later, was to bring his genius to bear on this brutalized human material and forge out of it the weapon that won the fields of Blenheim and Malplaquet, of Ramillies and Oudenarde, is a testimony as much to the native qualities of the soldiers as to the

---

* The quality of the officers may be judged by the fact that Colonel Luttrell's Regiment of Foot included a captain aged sixty-nine and two ensigns aged fourteen and twelve respectively.

giant stature of their leader. 'He was such a man,' said one veteran, 'that we forgot to be afeared.'

These were the men who came to occupy their village in Chelsea in the Spring of 1692. They brought with them their passion for alcohol and their lurid language. They also brought some primitive habits. Fox and Wren must have understood the problem, for the Instruction Book of 1692 gives these directions to the two Hospital sweepers, who rejoiced in the Dickensian names of Ciprian Whitwood and Thomas Winks:

> 'You are to admonish the soldiers *from time to time* (sic) not to throw any pieces of Tobacco, Pipes, foul Papers or Raggs into the Quadrangle Court nor into either of the Side Courts.'

It is not too difficult to imagine the quality of language that flowed from time to time between the In-Pensioners and Ciprian Whitwood and Thomas Winks. Nor did the old soldiers mend their ways, for in 1785, the Governor, Sir George Howard, addressed himself thus to Robert Adam, Clerk of the Works:

> 'I desire to draw your attention to the practice of Pensioners who do empty their personal soil and filth out of the Ward windows and under the walls leading to the Outer Courts. I further commend to your notice that it is the duty of the Sweepers to remove the same.'

From the top floor of the main wings to the courtyard there are six flights of stairs. It was a long way to carry chamber utensils.

From the outset the Royal Hospital was classed as a garrison and guards were mounted at the main gates until the middle of the last century. During the early years, In-Pensioners on guard duty were issued with short flintlocks, 'captains' carried half pikes, and sergeants the traditional halberd. The old men would not have provided very formidable opposition for their musketry days were over and the first three issues of ammunition were all found to be defective. Nonetheless the issue of arms gave a soldierly air to the place even if, on some ceremonial occasions, the procedure literally misfired. A visitor attending a military funeral in the Burial Ground recounted that when the order was given to the firing-party, some of the old men forgot the proper drill; whereupon they received

from their irate comrades a volley of such obscene language that
the shocked visitor fled for his life.

The firing-party was in action within ten days of the opening of
the Hospital, for on April 6 the first In-Pensioner was interred in
the Burial Ground. This was Simon Box, whose tombstone tells us
that he was 63 and had served four kings from Charles I to William
III, 'whose pentioner he was'. An examination of the muster rolls
suggests that he was a private of the Tangier Horse, later the 1st
Royal Dragoons, and that he had been severely wounded 'in Fight'.

The first action of Matthew Ingram, the Major, was to put the
In-Pensioners into a uniform dress more regimental and more
fitting to their new station than the interim clothing he had designed
for the Out-Pensioners. He struck upon the sensible solution of
fitting them out in ordinary cavalry or infantry uniforms according
to the arm in which they had served; and here we may conveniently
summarize the main details of these uniforms and the changes that
have taken place down to the present day. The old and the new are
illustrated on p. 111 and pp. 202–3.

In-Pensioners of the rank of corporal and below were initially
dressed thus:

'A *Red Cloth Coat* with Brass Buttons lined with blew Bays & False Sleeves, with a large Cypher of the King and Queen on the Back, And blew Kersey Breeches lined with brown Ossenbriggs.	£1	14	0
Two Black Hats with Copper Edgings & white hair hatbands at 5s. 6d. each		11	0
Two Pairs of Stockings at 1s. 7d. a pair		3	2
Two Pairs of Shoes at 4s. a pair		8	0
A Pair of Shoe Buckles			3
Four Shirts at 2s. 8d.		10	8
Four Neckcloths at 8d. each		2	8
Two Night Caps at 5d. each			10
	£3	10	7'

The higher ranks were distinguished by colour and quality. Thus
Sergeants of Foot and Light Horsemen wore a *Crimson Cloth Coat*,
gold braid, a more elaborate cocked hat and breeches of broadcloth
at a total cost of £5 19s. 3d. Curiously these grades were not issued
with shirts, neckcloths or night caps so presumably they were permitted some latitude in purchasing such items for themselves; and
predictably the cavalrymen at once objected to being classed with

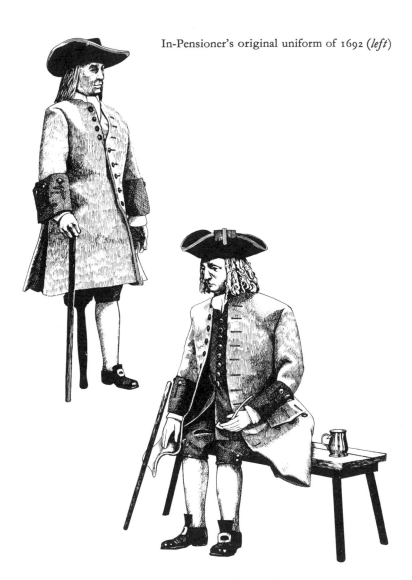

In-Pensioner's original uniform of 1692 (*left*)

In-Pensioner's 'Marlborough pattern' uniform of 1703

lowly Sergeants of Foot, for the latter were presently down-graded to silver braid, pewter buttons and less elaborate hats.

Finally the 'Captains' were dressed in a *Scarlet Cloth Coat* of superior quality, breeches of 'fine Blew Cloth', 'fine Blew stockings' and a cocked hat decorated with quantities of gold lace, at a total cost of £8 9*s.* 3*d.*

The clothing issue, known as the 'full mounting', was designed to last for two years, but some of the items, such as two shirts and one pair of shoes, were held back as replacements during the second year. As we shall see, In-Pensioners' kit soon became another fruitful source of beer-money.

In 1701, after ten years of partial eclipse, the Duke of Marlborough was appointed Commander-in-Chief. He inherited from William III an army greatly reduced in numbers and discontented to the point of mutiny. He alone understood the challenge this army would very shortly have to face and at once he set about rebuilding its pride and its morale. A clean soldier is a confident soldier and so Marlborough turned first to the re-equipping and re-clothing of his men, and in the directions he gave he did not forget the In-Pensioners at Chelsea.

On April 1, 1703 the Commissioners were instructed to enter into a new contract with 'Robert Cox, factor, of the City of London' for the issue of new uniforms for the Royal Hospital, including the twenty-four staff matrons and ten servants. The sealed patterns were virtually the same as those designed ten years earlier except for the addition of blue waistcoats and some distinctive embellishments, chiefly to gratify the fashion-conscious cavalrymen. The Commissioners drove a hard bargain. Not only was Robert Cox required to accept a contract price some 10 per cent lower than any previous quotation, but he was directed 'to deliver all the aforesaid items and accoutrements on or before May 27 next'; in other words the contract stipulated the delivery of 510 full mountings in *eight weeks* from the date of signature. Payment was to be made in equal quarterly instalments over a period of two years and since no accounts have survived, it is a fair assumption that Robert Cox was the only party to honour the contract. By 1708 he had been replaced – probably to his considerable relief – by another clothing contractor.

For nearly 140 years, the In-Pensioners' uniforms remained unchanged except for small and insignificant details, and thus the old soldiers must have appeared to the early Victorians as a quaint and even comical survival from another world. Indeed, by 1840 they had become such objects of ridicule that a drastic overhaul of Royal

Hospital dress was set in train.* Since these innovations have survived with only minor alterations to the present day, we may summarize the sequence of their introduction here:

1841. Blue trousers with scarlet piping. Ankle boots.

1842. The 'shako'-style forage cap bearing the letters R.H.

1850. The three-quarter length scarlet coat with blue collar and cuffs.

1859. A new pattern cocked hat priced at 5*s.* 6*d.* instead of 3*s.* 6*d.*

1868. The 'cheesecutter' cap worn by Hospital NCOs of the rank of Sergeant and above.

1894. The blue double-breasted 'button' waistcoat, worn with the 'shako' cap.

1921. The single-breasted waistcoat worn only within the Hospital, and the soft cap which alone bears the In-Pensioner's former regimental cap-badge.

Today the old distinctions of 'Captain' and Light Horseman survive in three ways. Hospital Warrant Officers and Sergeants wear the distinctive 'cheesecutter' cap; their scarlet coats are distinguished by gold braid on pocket flaps and cuffs; and they carry their *Hospital* badges of rank on their blue waistcoats. When walking out in scarlet, all In-Pensioners wear the badge of their highest *service* rank.

The variety and quality of clothing issued to the modern In-Pensioner would have made old Robert Cox sigh. The cost would have made him whistle. In 1973 the value of an In-Pensioner's full mounting was £156·32p; and a comparison of those items common to both periods is illuminating:

	1703	1973
Scarlet coat	£1 14*s.* 0*d.*	£23·17p
Cocked hat	5*s.* 6*d.*	£14·50p
Stockings/socks	1*s.* 7*d.*	32p
Shoes	4*s.* 0*d.*	£2·53p
Shirts	2*s.* 8*d.*	£2·08p
Neckcloths	8*d.*	15p

Put another way, *seven* In-Pensioners of 1703 could have been fully kitted out for the price of a single 1973 scarlet coat. We have come a long way.

* The blue winter greatcoat had replaced the single-breasted 'surtout' in 1830.

The first Standing Orders for the Royal Hospital were laid down by Matthew Ingram in his capacity as Major and Lieutenant-Governor. At a time when army discipline was draconian and punishment brutal, the code of conduct at Chelsea was surprisingly humane. This may have had something to do with the quasi-monastic origins of the place but more certainly it is a reflection of Ingram's wisdom and commonsense, for he was one of the few to understand that then, as now, the officers and staff of the Royal Hospital were the servants and not the masters of the In-Pensioners. And so he sought to create a happy village community.

His orders dealt chiefly with the duties of guards and sentinels and with ensuring that an intrusive public in no way disturbed the atmosphere of cloistered calm. With so many crippled and infirm men under his command, the risk of fire was a constant hazard and the regulations forbidding the use of open lights or candles in the Long Wards are the only section of Standing Orders heavily under-lined in his own hand. The old men were further invited to cultivate the virtue of cleanliness and were instructed in the need for vigilance against 'bugges and other vermin' in their quarters. Above all, the good Major was a fresh-air fiend and his orders required that windows should at all times be kept open during daylight hours.

Routine discipline was delegated to a duty 'Captain' who was instructed 'not to suffer any provisions to be sold in the Hall or near the Cupola [*elsewhere, presumably, it was a case of the survival of the quickest*], or any Disturbance to be made in the College Courts, or to see any Drunken Pensioners without sending them Prisoners to the Guard'. The Guardroom must have been kept busy as the tipplers came and went but apart from those cooling-off periods so dear to the hearts of all soldiers, the only forms of punishment seem to have been confinement to barracks and, as the ultimate sanction, dismissal from the Hospital. The first to go, according to the records, was In-Pensioner John Mullin who was 'turned out of the College for uttering a treasonable statement'. Since he was an Irishman, we may presume that he had been airing his Jacobite sentiments; and in that he was certainly not alone.

While Ingram attended to matters military, Fox and Wren, in accordance with the directions of the Royal Warrant, drew up a detailed Instruction Book which set out the duties and obligations of every member of the staff from Physician to Canal Keeper. These instructions tell us a great deal about the daily life of the Hospital, although the later archives suggest that they were more often

'Perfecere Gulielmus et Maria, Rex et Regina'

honoured in the breach than the observance. Here are some random samples:

To Augustin Frezer and Emanuel Langford, Chaplains:
'You are during your respective Wayteings to say prayers twice a day in the Chappell, vizt. Morning Prayer to begin constantly att Halfe an Houre after Tenn att furthest; and Evening Prayer att Halfe an houre after five from Lady Day to Michaelmas; And from Michaelmas to Lady Day att Halfe an Houre after Three.
You are to preach a Sermon every Sunday morning. . . .
You are to administer the holy sacrament of the Lords Supper att least Thrice in a year. . . .'

To Charles Fraiser, Phisitian
'You are frequently to visitt the sick and wounded and prescribe for their cure and Dyet, directing orders for their cure to the Chirurgeon or Apothecary and for their Dyett to the Housekeeper.
You are to notify your days of attendance at the said Hospital. . . .'

To Francis Beccles, Sexton
'You are not to suffer any Person whatsoever to sit upon the sixteen forms appointed for the soldiers, Nor to lett any Doggs come into the Chappel, nor women with Pattens.'

To John Grahme, Steward
'You are to buy and provide good and wholesome provisions for the Officer's Table in the Great Hall, taking care that the whole Expence of the said Table do not exceed Tenn shillings a day [*for sixteen persons*].
You are to have a strict eye to the Cookes . . . that no Embezzlement or Wast be committed by any of them.'

To Arthur Penn, Usher of the Hall
'You are to lett no body into the Hall when the Soldiers are at Dinner or Supper except the Officers and Servants of the Hospitall. But you may admitt any Body into the Gallery who desires to see them eat.'*

To John Hawkins, Wardrobe keeper
'You are to wait upon all Persons of Quality who wish to see the Hospital, and show them the Halls, Wards, Chappel, Walks, etc.'

* For some reason visiting the Great Hall during Pensioners' mealtimes was for many years a popular form of entertainment.

This Instruction Book was a model of its kind, framed to ensure efficient but unofficious management; but Fox and Wren had reckoned without the Earl of Ranelagh.

While his two colleagues were thus engaged in setting up the machinery of government for the Royal Hospital, Ranelagh continued to cultivate his garden at the public expense. He was not remotely interested in the welfare of the In-Pensioners whose arrival at Chelsea seemed like an unwarranted intrusion into his private affairs. Fox and Wren sought at all costs to avoid that head-on collision with him which would only have strengthened his position, and so their first step was to produce an estimate of the true cost of running the Hospital, based for the first time on actual figures rather than guesswork. This threw up a sum of £12,029 and on this basis Fox himself suggested that the old method of financing the Hospital out of the poundage fund and day's pay should be replaced by a fixed allocation amounting in all to about £15,000 a year. This proposal was accepted and incorporated in a Royal Warrant dated March 21, 1693 which also included two regulations designed to clip the Paymaster's expansive – and expensive – wings. It need hardly be added that within six months Ranelagh had found all the loop-holes he needed to evade these restrictions.

Rising costs, the embezzlement of catering funds, and the continued outlay on improvements to Ranelagh House soon created a new crisis in the Hospital's financial affairs and in order to effect economies, Ranelagh turned his guns on the pensioners. In the Spring of 1695, the pay of In-Pensioner 'Captains' was reduced from £9 2s. to £5 a year, that of Light Horsemen and Sergeants from £5 4s. to £4, and of private men from £1 15s. to £1. Nor was that all. From 1697 onwards, all payments to In-Pensioners were discontinued on the arbitrary authority of the Paymaster. Why Fox and Wren permitted this to happen is difficult to understand. The Governor, Sir Thomas Ogle, was too senile to notice, and Matthew Ingram, the soldiers' friend, was dead.

Ranelagh next turned his attention to the Out-Pensioners. The gentlemen of the Life Guards were reduced from 10s. 6d. a week to 7s.* and all rates except the lowest for Privates of Foot were cut

* They were accordingly known as 'King William's Seven Shilling Men.'

proportionately. And to ensure that the total cost was held down, the pension list was virtually closed to new admissions until, as we have seen, it reached the melancholy figure of fifty-one.

At the Committee of Inquiry in 1702 it was eventually discovered that no out-pensions had been paid since July 1, 1696 and that a sum of almost £5,000 was due to the old soldiers, most of which was owing to those trusting citizens of Westminster and Chelsea 'who have supported them (the Out-Pensioners) ever since the year 1696 in expectation of the said pensions, and are great sufferers, and some of them entirely impoverished thereby.' To us today it seems almost inconceivable that so great a scandal could have continued for so long; but it was a scandalous age in which the poor and impotent went to the wall, unnoticed and unwept.

At his examination, Ranelagh admitted that out-pensions for the years 1696–8 had only been paid in part and that he had withheld most of the sum of £5,300 advanced to him in November, 1698 for the purpose of discharging these debts. Such small amounts as he had paid to the landlords of the Out-Pensioners were, he confessed, simply in the nature of hush-money. One is almost inclined to admire his effrontery.

But the sands were running out for Richard Jones, Earl of Ranelagh. Astonishingly, the Royal Hospital had survived his seventeen years of undetected crime. After that, it could survive anything.

7
The Village comes of age

❧

An Interlude

It is 1702, and a convenient point at which to take stock; for on
December 7 of this year the Royal Hospital celebrated the twenty-
first anniversary of its foundation, and two weeks later finally rid
itself of the unwelcome attentions of Lord Ranelagh. It also saw the
end of the long partnership between Sir Christopher Wren and Sir
Stephen Fox for when, in February of the following year, the first
independent Board of Commissioners was appointed, Fox asked for
his name to be withdrawn. He was now 75 and after a life-time
spent in the public service, he might reasonably have sought a hard-
earned retirement. But the fact that he was appointed a Director of
Greenwich Hospital in July suggests that his resignation from the
Chelsea Board may have been coloured by his dislike of the new
Paymaster, Jack Howe. If this was so, then his judgement was to be
fully vindicated twelve years later.

The village was now complete, the buildings finished and the
gardens laid out and stocked. There was nothing in England to
compare with it for dignity and elegance. To Wren and Fox it must
have seemed something like a miracle. It had weathered three
reigns. It had survived a chronic shortage of money under Charles;
a Revolution under James; and the Earl of Ranelagh under William.
During the past five years the Treasury had three times given serious
consideration to the question of closing it down and indeed it
required only simple arithmetic to show the economies that could be
made by reverting its 476 occupants to out-pension. That it was
reprieved by the persuasive advocacy of Stephen Fox is beyond any
doubt. He had only to quote Ranelagh's disgraceful treatment of the
Out-Pensioners to show the fate of the old soldiers if they should be
'turned out of the house'. And despite – or perhaps because of – his
military preoccupations, King William stood firmly on the soldiers'
side. Besides, Fox could point to Wren's masterpiece, the Royal
Naval Hospital, now approaching completion at Greenwich.

Wren paid a private visit to Chelsea in April, 1702. He had a
particular affection for the place because he had built it not for kings

or princes, but for the old, the infirm, and the deserving. He spent that day talking to the In-Pensioners. We do not know how his conversations went, but he was now an old man among old men. He must have asked them if they were comfortable and if they had any complaints. And because they were old soldiers, they would certainly have found something to grumble about. The Pensioners may not even have known who he was, but they would have agreed with Thomas Carlyle when many years later he described the Royal Hospital as 'the work of a gentleman'.

When the Commons Committee met at the end of the year to examine Lord Ranelagh's conduct at the Pay Office, they were unable to inspect his accounts, for the excellent reason that no such accounts existed and the finances of the army in general and the Royal Hospital in particular were – not to put too fine a point upon it – confused. In fact, Ranelagh's accounts for the last four years of his stewardship were not passed until thirty-seven years later – and by Robert Walpole, who by then himself had some explaining to do.

On p. 120 is the balance sheet for the Royal Hospital over the entire period 1681 to 1702. These figures have been extracted from a detailed study of the relevant documents and had they been available to the Committee of Inquiry, it would have discovered that the Earl of Ranelagh had 'overspent' or, less delicately expressed, misappropriated the sum of £31,713 17s. 6¼d. When all those years later, this deficiency came to light, the books were balanced by a transfer from army accounts – which themselves had shown a deficiency of £72,000 over the period!

The remaining figures are self-explanatory and revealing, not least the modest total for 'land, building and furnishing'. For those with a nose for comparative costs, it may be of interest to record that the total bill for St Paul's Cathedral (where no land charge was involved) came to £738,845 5s. 2½d. By any standard, the Royal Hospital was a remarkable bargain.

So, as the new century begins, the Royal Hospital enters upon another phase in its long and chequered history. The next hundred years will show that Lord Ranelagh had no monopoly in the art of manipulating public money, and that where mismanagement and corruption were concerned, the seventeenth century had little to teach the eighteenth.

ROYAL HOSPITAL. BALANCE SHEET, 1681–1702

Receipts

	£	s.	d.	£	s.	d.
Poundage	366,372	1	10¼			
Poundage from officers' full and half pay	1,215	0	5½			
Sales of commissions	1,317	15	0			
Day's pay	23,232	5	9¾			
				392,137	3	1½
Legacies, etc.	13,775	5	3			
Transferred from army accounts	31,713	17	6¼			
				45,489	2	9¼

Total: £437,626 5 10¾

Expenditure

Chelsea Hospital	£	s.	d.	£	s.	d.
Land, building and furnishing	157,404	17	0¼			
Salaries, maintenance and every In-Pension charge	118,647	18	1			
Treasurer's salary and expenses	7,070	13	4			
				283,123	8	5¼
Other						
Out-Pensions	51,254	15	7½			
Pay Office, War Office, Exchequer fees	103,248	1	10			
				154,502	17	5½

Total: £437,626 5 10¾

8
Queen's pawns

❧

The long century that separates Blenheim from Waterloo is the most varied and colourful in the history of the Royal Hospital. During these hundred or so years, it began to develop a personality of its own and to fashion for itself a particular place in the mainstream of traditional English life. This was almost entirely due to the character of the In-Pensioners themselves, for they received precious little help from other quarters; on the contrary, they might well have echoed the old cynic's cry: 'With friends like these, who needs enemies?'

There is one aspect of this period which seems to have escaped previous historians of Chelsea and which we shall find illllustrated again and again throughout this chapter and the next. During these hundred years the Royal Hospital was two separate worlds, divided by a curious kind of social hypocrisy. Of the nine Governors between 1704 and 1815, only three troubled to occupy their official apartments. Two of them managed to combine their Chelsea appointment with the rather more time-consuming duties of Commander-in-Chief of the British army. One even succeeded in completing his period of office without once visiting the Hospital. It was the apotheosis of government by remote control.

The disease was catching. Further down the scale, the Hospital staff – and a good many people who had no connection with Chelsea – indulged in a private game of musical chairs. Patronage was the order of the day and even a modest place at the Hospital became a much sought-after prize, not out of any desire to be of service to the In-Pensioners but because it was a lucrative pastime. During his twenty-seven years as Clerk of the Works, Robert Adam – whose talents were worthy of a better occupation – spent a large part of his time on alterations and embellishments to officers' quarters and in gratifying the whims of what had become a village of social climbers. While the public at large enjoyed the elegant diversions of Ranelagh Gardens, a charmed circle savoured the private hospitality of the Governor's Table and the Festival Dinners; and in the best tradition of Lord Ranelagh himself, Sir Robert Walpole dipped his hand in the Chelsea till and built himself a suitably grand house on Hospital property.

Meanwhile, what of the In-Pensioners? Their world was very different. Between 1715 and 1806 not a penny of Hospital money was spent in improving their condition. Throughout those years their Long Wards were untouched except for running repairs. Their 'peculiar money' remained unchanged although by 1806 the value of the pound had been halved. Their diet, in theory unaltered except for the disappearance of fish in 1747, became in practice a happy hunting-ground for a succession of fraudulent Comptrollers and Master Cooks. At least they appear to have remained decently clothed.*

During this period they emerge for the first time from their early anonymity and we shall presently meet some of them and learn how they adapted themselves to this brave new world. They had all seen enough service to take corruption and inefficiency in their stride and they were wise enough in the ways of old soldiers to lead their superiors a merry dance; as, for example, In-Pensioner John Myland, of the 20th Foot, who installed his wife in the laundry and made a killing taking in the washing of the local gentry at cut prices.

It is a constantly shifting scene and we shall move from place to place as the wind of change blows.

But first we must take our final leave of the Earl of Ranelagh whose last – and literal – legacy to the Royal Hospital produced a situation of high comedy. In 1695, Ranelagh had made a settlement of £10,000 on his daughter, Frances. When three years later she married Lord Coningsby, her father – as a mark of his disapproval – set aside £3,250 from her dowry to be applied after his death for the benefit of the In-Pensioners. Since it is an entirely reasonable assumption that this money had been originally embezzled from Hospital funds, his Lordship's generosity was rather less than altruistic. When, in due course, he was faced by bankruptcy, Ranelagh made strenuous efforts to break the trust but not even his native ingenuity could persuade the Master of Chancery to subvert the law; and thus thwarted, Ranelagh directed that the income of £200 from the bequest should be applied for the provision of a 'surtout coat'† once every three years for each pensioner other than

---

* The cost of clothing In-Pensioners remained unchanged for fifty-three years, from 1708 to 1761, at an annual sum of £1,173 12s. 11d.

† At Ranelagh's death, a surtout coat cost £1. The figure today is £19·56. Accordingly they are now supplied from M.O.D. votes and the balance of income from the trust (around £250) is paid to the War Office. The wheel has come full circle.

'Captains' and Light Horsemen and that any surplus should be used annually to provide 'drink money' for all ranks on Founder's Day. In 1720, the legacy was subscribed into the South Sea Company and when that celebrated bubble burst it carried with it most of the late Lord Ranelagh's good intentions; whereupon the Master of the Rolls ordered that any deficiency should be made good out of another legacy of £2,000 which had been left to the Hospital in 1708 by John de la Fontaine. There the matter might have rested; but there was one last Gilbertian twist to come. When in 1742 the Commissioners started to purchase back the land conveyed fifty years before to the Earl of Ranelagh, their first acquisition was a parcel of three acres for which they paid £461 5s. – out of the Ranelagh legacy.

On February 6, 1703, two months after Ranelagh's resignation from the Pay Office, Queen Anne confirmed by Royal Warrant the appointment of the first independent Board of Commissioners for the Royal Hospital. Its members were: the Paymaster-General,* the Surveyor-General, the Paymaster in the Low Countries, and 'the Governor and Deputy Governor of the Hospital for the time being'. Behind this long overdue reform was the hand of the Commander-in-Chief, Marlborough, who a few months previously had introduced sweeping reforms in the administration of the Army. Not the least of these was a procedure designed to limit the powers of the Paymaster-General, who alone of the new Board was not permitted to sign warrants for any payments in connection with the running of the Hospital. It would be gratifying to think that this simple expedient finally laid the ghost of Ranelagh and ushered in an era of honest administration. Honesty, however, was not one of the sovereign virtues of the eighteenth century, in which the forms of corruption differed from those of the previous age only by their greater degree of sophistication and the richness of their harvest.

The new Paymaster-General was Jack Howe, a political firebrand with a well-exercised talent for opposition. His persistent criticism of William III must have commended itself to Queen Anne, for in 1702 he was made a Privy Councillor and his appointment to the

* Since this date the Paymaster-General has been , by virtue of his (or her) office, the Treasurer of the Royal Hospital and Chairman of the Board of Commissioners.

Pay Office followed six months later. He proved to be a good servant of the In-Pensioners, but he was a Whig among Tories and his long involvement in the political in-fighting of Anne's reign may have distracted him from the new scandals which shortly beset the Royal Hospital and which in due course drove him from public life.

The Surveyor-General was still Sir Christopher Wren, now in his seventies and greatly preoccupied with the building of St Paul's and of the new Hospital at Greenwich. With the retirement of Stephen Fox, he represented the last element of the old régime in the management of Chelsea. But a typical example of this extraordinary man's continuing attention to detail is to be found in the Chelsea Journal for May 29, 1707. On this date, the master-mason submitted an estimate for new paving in Figure Court (670 feet of Denmark stone at 3*d*. a foot!). Wren noted:

> 'The price seems reasonable if the work be directed to be done, and I am farther of the opinion that more than £1000 work be layd out in necessary repairs to prevent further Damages.'

There follows an estimate for repairing walks and stone steps, chimneys, paving in the Octagon porch, and paving in Light Horse and Infirmary Courts; building new chimney stacks; extensive work on the canals; and providing new railings. (All this despite the fact that the Hospital had only been opened fifteen years previously). Wren approved the total figure of £1,060 but carefully marked in the margin a list of first priorities amounting to £608.

The Paymaster in the Low Countries was Charles Fox, who had been in and out of office for twenty years. His new post was made entirely independent of Jack Howe and his scrupulous honesty and efficiency in paying the Army in the field contributed notably to the success of the Blenheim campaign.

The new Governor who succeeded Sir Thomas Ogle was Col. John Hales, a confirmed Jacobite, who owed his position to the Duke of Marlborough with whom he had been confined in the Tower in 1692. A few months before his appointment to the Royal Hospital he had been made Governor of Barbados and, in the spirit of the times, he retained that title – and its emoluments – for two years without once visiting his Caribbean parish; and, as we have seen, he contrived to continue for his own enjoyment the additional salary of £200 paid exclusively to Sir Thomas Ogle 'and not to any succeeding Governor'.

Finally, the office of Lieutenant-Governor on the new Board was filled by David Crauford, the first and last civilian to hold that post, in which, as Deputy Commissary-General of the Musters, he had succeeded Matthew Ingram in 1695.

At their first meeting on February 24, the new Board set about clearing out the Augean stables which they had inherited from Lord Ranelagh.

They turned first to the staff and, in a lengthy instruction, enjoined attention to duty, no absence without leave on pain of suspension, and promised continuity of employment for all officers and servants except for misdemeanour or abolition of office. They went on:

> 'No person (shall) be admitted an Officer or Servant in the said Hospitall but who have served in the Army and are not a Pensioner in the Hospitall. Allso that all the women Servants be widdows or wives of Soldiers not Pensioners in the said Hospitall.'

This admirable policy proved to be short-lived for within a few years most of the staff positions were occupied by unqualified civilians or their deputies and Hospital places were being bought and sold with a total disregard for regulations. It was not until Lord John Russell's reforms over a century later that the Board's directions were re-established. They have now lapsed once more.

Next, the Commissioners turned their attention to victualling. Two directives of March 3 and 6 laid down that the daily cost of the Governor's Table was not to exceed 13*s.* a day 'besides Bread and Beer', based on an average of sixteen persons to be so entertained. And the main contracts for provisions were renewed for one year on the following basis:

Butcher. To serve Beef and Mutton at two shillings and fourpence a Stone, nine pounds to the stone [*viz: 3d. a pound*].
Brewer. To serve 'fine drink' at one half penny a quart.
Baker. To serve Seventeen ounces of bread for one penny, to be made in fifteen ounce loaves.
Cheesemonger. To serve Cheese at three pence farthing a Pound and Butter at Fivepence half Penny a Pound.
Tallow Chandler. To serve Candles at five shillings and fourpence per dozen [*always a surprisingly expensive item*].

Having dealt with matters of physical welfare, the Board now addressed themselves to the subject of discipline. The stream of orders and directives which emerged over the following two years suggests that the Royal Hospital had become a very disorderly house, and indeed a local worthy, Jonathan Taylor, was shocked by 'the excesses which I did have occasion to observe when I was lately visiting the Colledge.' Here are two examples of the Board's instructions – one mysteriously vague, the other delightfully precise.

On April 10, 1703:

> 'Whatever appears to be a Newsance to the Hospitall shall be removed. The Governor and Clark of the Workes do view what has been built or sett up by Doctor Langford [*Augustine Frezer's successor as Chaplain*] to the Newsance of the House and direct that the same be pulled down.'

And on May 5, 1704:

> 'Whereas we are informed that the Under Butlers at the Royal Hospitall at Chelsea do make the Cellars in the said Hospitall a Tipling House for all comers and goers contrary to the Intention thereof, we doe hereby direct that the Steward and Comptroller of the said Hospitall do take care to prevent all Tipling in the said Cellars for the future and that if any seates or drinking places be set up, that they be immediately pulled down and removed. And that the Butler or any of his Deputies on any pretence whatsoever do not hereafter presume to sell any Ale, Beer, Brandy, Cyder, Port, Madeira or other liquors on any pretence whatsoever except to the Governor or to the Officers of the House, and that they shall not admitt any strangers whatsoever to drink in the Cellar under the Chapple nor suffer any music, singing or Smoaking in any of the Cellars belonging to the said Hospitall nor admitt of any drinking in the said Cellars in time of divine Service whether on Sundays or Weekdays.'

A visit to 'the said Cellars' today conjures up a smoky vision of merry-making and carousal, the sober chanting of the chapel choir punctuated by bawdy ditties from below. Nor does the Board's cautionary finger-wagging seem to have had much effect, for in 1728 In-Pensioner Rodenhurst was expelled from the Hospital for 'disgraceful and profane misconduct in the chappel cellar'.

We may pause here to consider for a moment one perennial aspect of Chelsea life. It was always a great place for tippling, partly because when two or three old soldiers were gathered together, it was sure to be over quarts of ale, and partly because the In-Pensioners had very little else to do. Until the nineteenth century there were no facilities for recreation at the Hospital and despite Evelyn's pious hopes, there was no library until 1823. As it was then run by the Chaplain, the choice of books must have been cautiously conservative. How the Pensioners managed to pay for their liquid diet is something of a mystery for even if they had spent their entire weekly subsistence of 8*d*. on beer, it would only have bought them at best 32 pints – scarcely a prescription for riotous living. We must assume that they supplemented their income by selling rations and clothing or, more probably, by trading old soldiers' tales and stories of misfortune in return for 'beer and baccy' in the local taverns. No Pensioner worth his salt would have gone unsatisfied for long.

Drinking seems to have been the curse of the Royal Hospital throughout the centuries and if we take the year 1763 as an example, of the thirty-six men 'turned out of the House', thirty-one went on their way because of persistent drunkenness; and if we look at some of their names – Sullivan, Mahon, Donnellon, Rorke – we can draw at least one conclusion! The problem remained until the opening of the In-Pensioners' Club in 1952 when decent facilities removed most of the incentives for over-indulgence.

It was not long before the Hospital was again in serious financial difficulties – although this time the reasons were more complex and intractable.

The Board's first task was to clear the out-pension arrears of £5,000 dating back to 1696, most of which, as we have seen, was paid to the long-suffering citizens of Westminster and Chelsea who had billeted the old soldiers at ruinous cost to themselves.

But this was a very temporary palliative; and within two years out-pensions had again fallen into arrears. The situation was aggravated by the growing cost of the war, by the resulting increase in men qualified for the pension list, and by the bitter political feuding which characterized Queen Anne's reign. On March 25, 1705, a few months after Blenheim, the Board drew the attention of Henry St John, then Secretary at War, to the fact that of the wounded men returning from Germany and Holland '41 with running wounds have been taken into the Hospital and the rest ordered into quarters'.

The Board pointed out that there was no money available for the latter, that 'most of them are very ill cloathed and will be quite naked before they can come into ye Hospital'; and requested a fund for clothing them and paying their quarters at a rate of 2*s.* a day 'which we think as low as the businesse can be performed'.

Six days later, Wren, Fox and Crauford informed Godolphin, the Lord High Treasurer, that a special bounty of £4,000 provided by Charles Fox out of his separate funds was insufficient to meet the bill and asked for additional money (£2 10*s.* a man for clothing and 10*s.* a man for those discharged to their homes). Somewhat tardily, their request was met out of the Exchequer Vote.

We may digress for a moment here to consider the plight of the Out-Pensioners. In spite of the original Royal Warrant of 1685 (renewed with two minor variations by Queen Anne in 1709), they were treated with a cynical disregard for their welfare (it was not until 1806 that they had any *rights*). Throughout the early part of the century they were used first as a political counter and then as a stalking-horse for every corrupt practitioner who could squeeze a few pennies out of them. How they survived in a world where their pensions were constantly in arrears, savagely reduced, or never paid at all is a mystery. Many must have perished and others turned in desperation to crime. It is difficult to understand why they were still continued as a charge on Royal Hospital funds, since between 1702 and 1714 no less than £148,000 was paid by Exchequer Votes to rectify a generation of abuses. The likely answer is that the administration of army funds, the obvious source for the payment of out-pensions, was subject to even greater abuse and inefficiency. The Earl of Lincoln, for example, who succeeded Robert Walpole as Paymaster-General in 1715, not only speculated privately with Hospital funds in the South Sea Company and lost nearly £7,500 as a result, but on his dismissal in 1720 found himself unable to account for the tidy sum of £473,000 out of monies provided for the Army.

It says much for the old soldiers that they endured so long in the face of such contempt and humiliation. They were now to need all their patience and fortitude.

Jack Howe soon found himself swimming against the tide, for as political temperatures rose, his relationship with the Chelsea Board and with his Tory opponents outside became increasingly strained. The argument was one of means rather than ends. The increasing cost of out-pensions continued to outrun the Hospital revenue and Robert Harley, the chief minister throughout most of this period, could see no political mileage in promoting the welfare of old or crippled soldiers. Howe accepted the need for retrenchment but not at the expense of human dignity. He repeatedly urged that the Hospital staff, swollen by patronage and wastefully inefficient, should be ruthlessly pruned. His suggestions, submitted in a series of caustic memoranda, were shelved or ignored. But on one point he was adamant: the In-Pensioners were the first charge on the available revenue and nothing was to be done that might adversely affect their interests. The old men were probably unaware of the argument raging around their heads, but since rumour was – and still is – part of the staple diet of Chelsea, they must have had a fair idea who was fighting their battle for them.

Unfortunately for Howe, he was not master in his own house. Until 1706, all admissions to the Royal Hospital were personally authorized by Marlborough, but since the Captain-General was occupied elsewhere, an order was issued on May 6 to the effect that 'Out-Pensioners may be taken into ye Hospital and In-Pensioners removed to ye Out-Pension at the discretion of the Governor.' Given a man of Col. Hales's character, it was a licence to commit nameless injustices; and the admission rolls indicate that he took full advantage of it.

There was another situation of which the Governor also took advantage, although in so doing he was unwittingly writing his own notice of dismissal. We last left the aged 'Catalogue' Fraser comfortably installed in his Hospital apartment, surrounded by his books and happily delegating his duties as Secretary and Register to his clerk. This clerk, by name James Crispe, was now given the full authority of his master's office by Hales. We do not know the precise nature of the deal they struck between them, but we may draw our own deductions from the fact that the cost of provisions rose from £4,930 in 1708 to £7,629 in 1712, despite the fact that the In-Pensioner establishment had fallen by four and the victualling contracts had been continued each year at identical and fixed rates. It is not without significance that the Board Minutes (kept by Crispe) for the years 1709 to 1711 are the only ones which have not survived.

The irregularities at Chelsea must have become common knowledge, for in 1711 an inquiry was conducted by the Commissioners of Accounts and although its findings have been lost, we know that proceedings were instituted against a number of 'the officers of Chelsea Hospital'. Among these was James Brydges, the future

Duke of Chandos and patron of Handel, who had succeeded
Charles Fox as Paymaster in the Low Countries in 1705, though not
on the Chelsea Board. Brydges was found guilty of having appropriated £6,000, representing five years' arrears due to the Royal
Hospital in respect of 'poundage and day's pay of the Forces under
his care', and in January 1712 he submitted his resignation, which
was not accepted. Instead, his punishment (*o tempora, o mores!*) was
to be appointed a Chelsea Commissioner.

As a result of the inquiry, £60,000 was voted for the Royal
Hospital to meet its various arrears. It seemed generous – except for
the fact that the arrears had accumulated to a total of *£84,000*, and
Howe was accordingly authorized to make up the deficit out of
Army funds. At the same time, he recommended a complete revision
of the Chelsea Board to include the Captain-General (now James
Ormonde, grandson of the great Duke) and a large contingent of
financial pundits, but excluding the Governor and his deputy. But
Howe had reckoned without Hales's influence in high places and
when the new Board was reconstituted* on February 23, 1712, both
he and David Crauford were reappointed. Howe's reply was to
boycott the new Board and although he continued to carry out his
Pay Office duties, he attended no more meetings until his resignation
two years later.

From the outset, Howe was now opposed by a powerful Jacobite
clique led by Ormonde, whose declared aim was to slash the cost of
the Royal Hospital or, if they could not achieve that end, to close it
down completely. Predictably they started with the Out-Pensioners
and in September Howe was instructed to cease all payments pend-
ing re-examination for the pension list. At the same time Ormonde
directed the Governor to admit seventy-four seriously wounded or
blind old soldiers to the Hospital, which necessitated the removal of
forty-seven In-Pensioners, half of whom were then refused entry to
the pension list.

Howe continued to remonstrate that the correct target should be
the Hospital staff 'where there are many unnecessary expenses and
abuses', but since most of his adversaries were themselves deeply
implicated in those very abuses, his advice fell on deaf ears.

Early in 1713, all Out-Pensioners were re-examined and 1,882
were struck off the list, leaving 1,719. It was a cynical and – as it
proved – futile exercise, but worse was to follow. From June 24 all

* The 1712 Board numbered fifty-six, including thirty-three Privy Councillors,
the Archbishop of York and the Bishop of London, none of whom put in an
appearance after the first meeting.

out-pensions were reduced to a flat rate of 5*d.* a day irrespective of rank, and were so continued with two minor exceptions until William Windham's Act of 1806. For this arbitrary action, no Royal Warrant exists. At the same time the pension list was closed to further admissions and the qualifications were restricted to 'wounds of exceptional gravity or thirty years unbroken service'. The effect of these draconian measures was to reduce the out-pension charge from £50,000 to £15,000 a year. It was a shabby economy, and five months later mounting indignation in army circles compelled Ormonde to re-instate all the Out-Pensioners he had struck off earlier in the year.

One consequence of the June 24 measures was a further vote of £60,000 to pay off accumulated arrears and this money was entrusted to Howe. Either through instinct or inside knowledge, he elected not to distribute it to the pensioners. It was to prove a wise decision.

On October 5, 1714, Jack Howe resigned from the Pay Office on grounds of ill-health, although he continued to act as Hospital Treasurer until the Spring of 1715. Within a week of his appointment, his successor, Robert Walpole, was asked by the Treasury Commissioners to investigate the state of affairs at Chelsea, and he invited Howe to submit a report on the subject. This memorandum, dated November 20, is a remarkable document for it is indirectly a self-indictment. Some weeks earlier, Howe had been instructed to obtain a nominal roll of the 1,719 Out-Pensioners remaining after the recent reduction, indicating the regiment and the qualification of each man, duly certified by the various officers concerned. Howe goes on:

'Instead thereof is lately sent me a book with eight thousand nine hundred and eighty* men's names, signed at the end by five Commissioners, without any distinction of the regiments or companies wherein they serv'd, or any account of their qualifications. . . . This book itself is not so much as paged, and has so many blank sides, besides other vacant places, that such a latitude is given for inserting so many more names than the Commissioners did actually sign to, as is not credible but by a view of it.'

A strong hint in the direction of James Crispe, now the acting Secretary and Register, is underlined by a barbed reference to the unexplained increase in the cost of provisions and 'contingencies' referred to previously. Howe then does some arithmetic for the

* Howe's arithmetic was wrong. The true total was 9,109.

Treasury Board in which he costs out the annual charge for the Royal Hospital, based on these discrepancies, and comes up with an excess of expenditure over income of £69,500. That he himself was the Paymaster-General at the time seems to have escaped him.

Armed with this memorandum, a Committee of the Privy Council was set up in January, 1715 to investigate the 'abuses and mismanage ments of the Royal Hospital near Chelsea.' The Committee pulled no punches in its report. 'There seems,' it observed drily, 'to be no discipline or regularity in any part of the management of the hospital.' It was the understatement of the year. Step by step the report uncovered the malpractices in the administration of pensions and the growing 'protection' racket to which the unfortunate Out-Pensioners had been subjected. And the 9,109 names in Jack Howe's dubious pay-book? Here the Committee is acid. 'Another advantage these persons seem to have, a man is no sooner admitted an invalid but he becomes immortal, there not having *one man* died out of 9,109, from the time of their first admission.'

Crispe, confronted with the evidence of the fraudulent pay-book, admitted nothing, but Butler Noades, the Surgeon's Mate, who had collaborated in the plot, finally confessed and in so doing implicated his accomplice. The Committee's finding was that of 'a scandalous remissness in the principal officers, and notorious corruption in the inferior, countenanced, if not encouraged, by the acting Commissioners.'

Jack Howe had already resigned; Col. Hales and David Crauford were dismissed from office; and Crispe and Noades, the only two culprits to be found guilty of malpractice, were arrested. In the event, no action was brought against them and they were subsequently released. For this they could probably thank Jack Howe's inspired decision not to release his £60,000 of out-pension money to the acting Secretary and Register. For once a public scandal had not ended in financial disaster.

With the removal of all the effective Commissioners, a new Board was constituted in March, 1715 under Robert Walpole, the Paymaster-General, and graced in name, if not in person, by the Duke of Marlborough, now restored to favour. The In-Pensioners could breathe again. Under a German King, perhaps the future might be different.

It was.

9
Characters grave and gay

❦

'G—— d—— King George for a Presbyterian S of a ——,
& I pray God send K ——
James ye third before Christmas
to injoy his Crown.'

For these unequivocal sentiments, coyly expurgated in the Chelsea
Board Minutes, In-Pensioner Hammett was expelled and 'turned off
the Pension' in September, 1716. Nor were such sentiments un-
representative of the attitude of many old soldiers on the accession
of Hanoverian George I, rooted as they were in a native dislike of
foreigners in general and foreign kings in particular. It had been
so in William III's time when the memory of the glorious Revolution was still fresh, and it persisted long after the abortive rising of
1715. The Chelsea archives bear witness not only to the strength of
Jacobite sympathies at the Royal Hospital but among those many
Out-Pensioners who, with an English lack of logic, held the new
régime responsible for the pension scandals of the previous reign.
It was by no means a universal sentiment, but the romantic notion
of 'the King over the water' died hard, and as late as 1761 Sergeant
Horton of the first Ward 'was broke and turned entirely off the
Pension for Treasonable Expressions against his Majesty' – a
punishment like that of In-Pensioner Hammett and, before him,
In-Pensioner Mullin.

For the most part, however, the old soldiers had long since
learned that discretion was the better part of valour. Not many
people cared about them, for in eighteenth-century England the
race was to the slickest and Georgian society was more concerned
in private gamesmanship than in social justice. The Out-Pensioners
continued to be ruthlessly exploited both by officialdom and by the
moneylenders who haunted the purlieus of the Royal Hospital; and
forty more years were to pass before the root cause of these abuses
was tackled, though even then the removal of one grievance was
replaced by another.

The decision to reduce all pensions to a flat rate of 5d., however,
had occasioned great distress and in the face of much agitation, a
new pension grade known as 'lettermen' was introduced in April,

133

1715. This grade, individually confirmed by royal letter, was restricted to those ranks which had previously qualified for 12*d*. a day, and this former rate was granted again in the first instance to an arbitrary selection of forty 'gentlemen' and cavalry sergeants (one tenth of the number entitled). In 1718 the figure was increased to 100 and in 1723 an intermediate grade of 9*d*. a day was introduced for the curious total of thirty-one sergeants of Horse Grenadiers and sergeants of the Guards. The 'lettermen' were subsequently increased again – to 200 in 1778 and to 400 in 1784, at which figure they remained until the grade was abolished by Windham's Act of 1806.

Meanwhile, back at the Hospital the In-Pensioners found their services in demand in an unexpected way. The road from Westminster to Chelsea had long been a favourite haunt of footpads for it was little more than a country lane passing through open fields and frequented for the most part by persons of quality. In 1715 it was also the road by which Robert Walpole returned to his lodgings at the Royal Hospital and he was probably the moving spirit behind a Royal Warrant addressed to the Governor in September of that year. This Warrant required the Governor 'to cause such a Number of Invalids belonging to Our Royal Hospital near Chelsea to be drawn out as shall be sufficient to patrole between Our Palace of St James's and Chelsea Town aforesaid, which patrole is to continue (from sunset) until 12 a Clock every night, and then to return to Our Royal Hospital.'

When this instruction duly appeared in orders, it must have occasioned some very choice language, but since the Hospital was classified as a Garrison, its inmates were liable for military duties. A patrol was duly formed consisting of two sergeants, four corporals and twenty 'private centinels', on a 'day on, day-off' basis. Any mutinous feelings were probably assuaged by the granting of extra-duty pay of 2*s*., 1*s*. 6*d*. and 1*s*. a week respectively, according to rank, and even the the simplest 'private centinel' could calculate that this bonus would buy 24 quarts of beer.

The old men paraded with 'muskets with Bayonets fix'd' and wore protective 'watch gowns' against the cold and wet. But they were thin on the ground and within a few months the patrol was attacked and one pensioner died of his injuries. Accordingly their number was increased by six and a guard-house was built at Ebury Farm (near the present Ebury Square) with sentry boxes at 300-yard intervals. It made little difference. Robbery with violence continued unabated, although the pensioners managed to claim some scalps (on at least one occasion the Chelsea patrol itself turned footpad), and it was not until a hundred years later that this useless exercise was discontinued. By then the introduction of street lighting and Fielding's Bow Street Runners had proved a more effective deterrent.

The period of this chapter is rich in 'characters', for the Hospital presently began to attract all sorts and conditions of men, some drawn there for good and innocent reasons, others – and they were more numerous – with less creditable intentions. Together they give this century its special flavour and we will examine some of the more notorious, beginning with the 'Chelsea Monarch' himself, Robert Walpole.

Walpole had first made his mark in public life in 1708 as Secretary at War in succession to the 'brilliant, fugitive rascal', Henry St John. Massive in bulk, gourmand and *bon viveur*, he was a Norfolkman and spoke like one, boasting that at table he 'always talked bawdy because in that all could join'. For twenty-one years, until his resignation in 1742, he presided over a nation at peace (the brief War of Jenkins's Ear was a minor ripple in a millpond), his political weapons a masterly use of moderation, financial expertise, and the ruthless management of Crown patronage. Under George I he had 'governed with bad Latin', for the King spoke no English and Walpole had neither French nor German. Subsequently, he skilfully manipulated Queen Caroline, the gouty but formidable consort of George II, and so complete was his domination of the political scene that he became in fact, if not in name, the first British Prime Minister. The Royal Hospital, however, has cause to remember him with something less than affection.

In 1712, Walpole had been briefly committed to the Tower by his inveterate enemy, the Tory Robert Harley, on a charge of embezzling £1,000 of public money. This accusation was in fact a by-product of the Commission of Inquiry into the financial conduct of the Duke of Marlborough who, under long-standing precedent, had received some £63,000 from the bread and transport contractors in the Netherlands together with a subvention of £280,000 for the Allied Secret Service fund. The allegations against the Commander-in-Chief were not substantiated, but enough mud stuck to bring about his resignation and that of his Whig adherents. Historians are unanimous in acquitting Walpole of the same charges, but his subsequent conduct, not least at Chelsea, argues otherwise.

With the accession of George I and the resignation of Jack Howe, Walpole was appointed to the Pay Office. His first tour of duty there lasted a year, his second – from June 17, 1720 – ten months, when in the chaos following the South Sea Bubble scandal he took office as Chancellor of the Exchequer and Chief Minister.

His passion for patronage was soon in evidence. Within a few days he had appointed as Deputy Treasurer of the Royal Hospital Robert Mann, an old crony and distant relative, who had been implicated in the charges which had landed Walpole in the Tower. In the following year he placed another of his protegés, Kingsmill Eyre, as acting Secretary and Register and on the compulsory retirement of 'Catalogue' Fraser in 1718, Eyre succeeded to the post. These distasteful creatures happily milked the Out-Pensioners under their master's nose for upwards of twenty-five profitable years (Kingsmill Eyre was subsequently found to have collected over £1,400 a year in illicit fees) and the Chelsea accounts bear witness to the range and versatility of their corruption.

But the 'Chelsea Monarch' had by no means finished. The position of Surgeon's Mate, left vacant by the removal of Butler Noades, was given to William Hepburn, nephew of his personal physician in Norfolk, and the new separate appointment of Master Baker went improbably to a Member of Parliament, Henry Parsons, who secured from Walpole not only the bread contract, but also those for meat, butter and cheese which reputedly brought him in a net rake-off of £500 a year, after rendering unto Caesar Caesar's due percentage. And while the flesh prospered, so did the spirit, for two of Walpole's nominees, Henry Bland and William Barnard, both notorious pluralists, occupied – largely *in absente* – the chaplaincy of the Hospital. It was worthwhile being a Whig.

Meanwhile Walpole was not idle in his own interest. On his arrival at the Pay Office, he at once addressed himself to the matter of accommodation. Ranelagh House was, of course, no longer the property of the Royal Hospital and was occupied by the late Earl's spinster daughter Catherine, who lived there in solitary state, mourning the demise of her inseparable companion, Mary Kendall, now five years dead and buried obscurely, if surprisingly, in West-

minster Abbey. We may remember that many years previously
Ranelagh's partner in crime, William Jephson, had acquired the
lease of four and a half acres on the western boundary of the Hospital
and there he had built himself a small house in Wren's stableyard.
At his death, the Crown lease was purchased by the first Earl of
Orford who had been First Lord of the Admiralty under Queen
Anne until his removal by Harley and St John. Jephson's house had
been duly appropriated by Jack Howe in his capacity as Hospital
Treasurer, and Orford's efforts to regain possession of the property
were brusquely rejected by the Chelsea Board.

The Treasurer's lodgings were much too modest for Walpole's
taste and he at once commissioned Sir John Vanbrugh, who had
combined the varied talents of soldier, dramatist and architect, to
carry out extensive alterations. These entailed the appropriation—
and removal – of various small dwellings which Wren had built for
humble members of the Hospital staff and the acquisition of most
of Jephson's original leasehold in conjunction with his next-door
neighbour, Sir Richard Gough. The following year, during his brief
occupancy of the Treasury, Walpole used – or abused – his position
to obtain a Crown lease* of thirty-one years for his new lodgings
on precisely the same terms which had been rejected in the case of
Lord Orford.

By the time it was finished, Walpole House, as it came to be called,
was virtually a new mansion; nor did matters end there. In the
spacious grounds, Vanbrugh built a greenhouse where Walpole
entertained his distinguished guests, and an L-shaped Orangery
which within the last few years has been beautifully restored to
house the Hospital library and a Roman Catholic oratory. Finally on
the river bank Vanbrugh designed a charming octagonal summer-
house with a Baroque cupola surmounted by a golden pineapple
and here, too, in this elegant setting Walpole wined and dined his
royal visitors. Nor was Lady Walpole excluded from all this architectural activity for she built herself a celebrated grotto in the area
where Gordon House now stands, an absurd eighteenth century
folly decked out with shells, coloured stones and little mirrors.

Time deals harshly with human vanities and today only Vanbrugh's Orangery has survived the march of progress.

Long after he had left the Pay Office for the loftier corridors of
power, Walpole continued to occupy his Chelsea house. It had cost

* To avoid any awkward questions, the lease was granted to Walpole's protegé
Kingsmill Eyre, who promptly reassigned it to his master for £1 – and 'divers
other good Causes and Consideracŏns'.

him nothing for, treading faithfully in the footsteps of Lord Ranelagh, he had appropriated the necessary money out of Hospital funds and Robert Mann, who held the purse-strings, had a vested interest in his master's continuing patronage. So much for history's verdict on this 'honest' broker. Even after moving into 10, Downing Street, of which complete with mistress, he was the first official occupant, Walpole conducted most of the affairs of state from Chelsea; and Queen Caroline, Regent during her husband's long absences a broad, dutifully attended upon her Chief Minister there.

So far as the In-Pensioners, and indeed the Royal Hospital, were concerned, they might as well not have existed. Not once are they mentioned in Walpole's lengthy private correspondence. Not once after 1721, does his name appear in the Board Minutes. For twenty-one years the 'Chelsea Monarch' reigned supreme and aloof, pausing only to feather his expensive nest out of the 'noble charity' next door. He should have done better, for at his death he left debts of £40,000.

Meanwhile on the other side of the Hospital, a very different kind of charade took place after Walpole's decline and fall in 1742.

In 1730, the Ranelagh estate had been vested in trustees and three years later the property was auctioned off with the exception of three acres on the south side of Light Horse Court which the Chelsea Commissioners, as we have seen, repurchased for £461.

Early in 1741, a speculative builder named Timbrell, who had already illegally erected at least one house on ground adjoining the old mansion, entered into partnership with Lacy, patentee of Drury Lane Theatre, to build a Rotunda or 'Musick Theatre' near Ranelagh House. Under the terms of the original lease, the Chelsea Board were perfectly at liberty to forbid any development which they considered detrimental to the interests of the Hospital, but despite their protests, this massive pleasure-dome, ingeniously designed by William Jones and constructed entirely of wood, was opened in April 1742. One hundred and eighty-five feet in diameter and eighty feet high, not much smaller than the Albert Hall, it must have towered over the near-by Hospital buildings. But Henry Pelham, the then Paymaster-General, was more interested in his political future than in the welfare of old soldiers, and thus the Board duly acquiesced in the vendors' proposals. More foolishly, they agreed to determine the nominal annual rent of £5 a year which Ranelagh had negotiated fifty years before, and thereby lost all future control in the development of his estate. Another eighty-five years were to elapse before the whole property returned to the Royal Hospital fold.

Ranelagh Gardens were the ultimate expression of the eighteen century passion for novelty. The Rotunda itself was the centrepiece lit by a thousand candles and decorated with paintings, and with discreet alcoves for the amorous or simply the hungry, and it stood in a setting of formal and informal gardens, Italianate, Chinese and English, with fairylit trees and an ornamental canal. Here, for the admission price of 1s., came the world and his wife, irrespective of class or station, although in due course the gentry took to arriving late when 'persons of inferior birth', who had to rise early for work, might be thought to have gone home to bed.

It was a place for music – Mozart, then aged eight, performed on the harpsichord in public – and dancing; but chiefly it was a place to see and be seen and most of the visitors merely perambulated aimlessly round the Rotunda. 'There are,' observed Dr Johnson drily, 'many happy people here . . . who are watching hundreds, and who think hundreds are watching them.'

After the bankruptcy of the first proprietors, Ranelagh Gardens achieved their finest hour under the imaginative direction of Sir Thomas Robinson. They were patronized by royalty, by everybody who was anybody – and by many who were nobody. Fanny Burney's *Evelina* was enchanted by the place. So was the effeminate Horace Walpole, who 'went every night constantly to Ranelagh' and indulged his waspish talent for epigram at the expense of both royalty and aristocracy. Chesterfield used it as his postal address, Joshua Reynolds and David Garrick attended a special gala, and Thomas Arne was director of music for many years. There were masked balls, firework displays, and on one exciting occasion, a balloon ascent. Tea, coffee, punch and wine were the usual refreshments (those with stronger stomachs probably frequented 'the Ginn shop at the end of the Burying ground') and a recently unearthed cache of hundreds of oyster shells reflects one facet of the public appetite.

But public taste is a fickle thing. By the turn of the century, the popularity of Ranelagh, as well as its standards of behaviour, had declined in the face of competition from Vauxhall across the river. In 1803, it opened its doors for the last time and two years later both Ranelagh House and the Rotunda were pulled down. It had always been a curious neighbour for the Royal Hospital. So far as one may judge, the thousands who flocked there paid little or no attention to Wren's 'stately fabrick' next door. Nor was the place frequented by the In-Pensioners, for in none of the many illustrations and engravings of Ranelagh do they feature at all. The sound of music and revelry until the small hours must have been a constant source of irritation to the old soldiers in their Long Wards, and those who may have been tempted to venture there in search of a free drink probably settled for 'the Ginn shop at the end of the Burying ground' instead.

While Walpole indulged himself on one side of the Hospital, and high society on the other, life in the village continued 'at a foot-pace'. As we look back through the archives and listen to the distant echoes, the picture grows sharper, the sounds more distinct. Each part of the village has its own, different story to tell; and since those who came here sought a refuge from age and infirmity, we will turn first to that side of village life which ministered to the old and the sick.

The first establishment for the Hospital had included a 'Phisitian' and a 'Chirurgeon', the former position filled by Charles Fraiser and the latter by John Noades, who had been a Regimental Surgeon in the Foot Guards, Judging by their relative salaries, the Physician was considered the senior appointment, understandably so since the practice of surgery was still a crude and primitive science in the late seventeenth century. Nonetheless the 1692 Instruction Book, while setting out the physician's duties, carefully glossed over those of the surgeon – and of the Apothecary who was, in effect, the resident medical superintendent. This lack of precise definition of responsibilities led in due course to considerable professional jealousy and, eventually, to a Gilbertian situation over salaries; but it was not until 1832 that the two appointments were merged under the present title of Physician and Surgeon.

The office of Apothecary was for fifty years the monopoly of the Garniers, a family of naturalized Huguenots, and it was for the first of them, Isaac, that Wren built his little 'Elabritory'. Here Isaac Garnier not only dispensed his potions, but fixed his prices. In-Pensioners then, as now, received free medical treatment and the Apothecary's charges were met out of Hospital funds. With a Frenchman's commercial instinct, Garnier in his first year made a clear profit of £200 to supplement his modest salary of £50, and when we look at his accounts – 'For Serjeant Burnett, a purging Potion 1/6d. For David Jones, a Bottle Elixir Salutis, 2/–' it is not difficult to see why the Garniers kept this lucrative occupation in the family.

Wren's Infirmary had been designed to provide thirty-two beds and, given the physical condition of many of the In-Pensioners, it was seriously under-equipped. It must therefore have been necessary to treat a considerable number of old men in their wards. This was particularly so during Marlborough's wars when the Commander-in-Chief directed that priority was to be given to battle casualties returning from the Low Countries. The Infirmary had never been intended to serve as a military hospital and in order to provide more beds, the least infirm among the In-Pensioners were summarily turned out on the streets. Since most of them were too old or crippled to earn a living and since out-pensions had by then become a lottery, they suffered greatly and in 1708 four such men are known to have died of starvation. It was rough justice indeed.

Throughout the eighteenth century the medical records of the Royal Hospital are very scanty. This is partly due to the haphazard standards of diagnosis and partly to the incomprehension of the members of the Chelsea Board. Neither the Physician nor the Surgeon attended meetings – indeed the Physician for many years rarely attended the Hospital. But a layman reading the Board Minutes must be struck by two constantly recurring medical themes: insanity and rupture.

To take a single year at random, in 1769 twenty-two In-Pensioners were committed to the asylum at Hoxton. Some of these cases were no doubt correctly diagnosed, but since the study of geriatrics was as yet unknown, it is more probable that these men were simply suffering from senility or from other emotional disturbances of the very old. But there is more sinister evidence in the Board Minutes that Hoxton was also used as a convenient dumping-ground for compulsive drinkers and even for pensioners who were simply unco-operative or 'difficult'. For such men – and Hoxton vied with Bedlam as a repository of the damned – it was a grisly punishment.

The extraordinary number of rupture cases is more understandable and the Hospital must have become a trussmaker's paradise. There are dozens of solemn references to the provision of 'trusses of a new and attractive (sic) pattern' or to 'an ingenious new appliance strongly recommended by Mr Ranby.' And thereby hangs a tale.

Sometime in 1750, Samuel Lee, a *soi-disant* surgeon practising in

Pimlico, asked for permission to experiment on a number of volunteer In-Pensioners with a new 'cure' for rupture. The then Surgeon of the Hospital refused, so Lee by-passed the authorities and treated eight old men privately; and a year later he presented the Hospital Treasurer with a bill for £265 8s. A heated correspondence ensued until – probably in sheer desperation – a high-powered medical Board was convened to examine Lee's curative claims. It did not take them long to dissect his dubious reputation. The Board Minute continues:

> 'Mr Lee then withdrew and meeting in the Waiting Room Mr Thomas, the Deputy Surgeon of the Hospital, he without any provocation gave to the said Mr Thomas in the presence of several persons very abusive, horrid and threatening language.'

That, however, was not quite the last of this egregious quack. Two months later he asked for a personal hearing for, so the Board Minute tells us, 'he had something material to say relating to some of the poor Pensioners. He was accordingly admitted. He then said he came to know the cause why several Men were turned out of the House. At which,' says the notably restrained Minute, 'the Commissioners ordered him to withdraw.'

The first great Surgeon of the Royal Hospital was William Cheselden, father of modern surgery, teacher and preceptor of John Hunter who worked and studied under him for two years at Chelsea, and celebrated for his 'lateral operation for the stone' which he was said to have been able to perform almost painlessly in 54 seconds. He has also been credited, probably apocryphally, with removing an In-Pensioner's gall-bladder under an anaesthetic of rum and laudanum.

Cheselden spent the last fifteen years of his distinguished career at the Hospital and at his death he was succeeded by John Ranby of whom it was said that 'his tongue was sharper than his surgeon's knife'. Ranby had seen active service and had written a standard work on the treatment of gunshot wounds and to that extent he could claim a specialist qualification for the Chelsea post. But he is best remembered in medical history as the first Master of the Company of Surgeons, formed by Cheselden in 1745 and destined in due course to become the Royal College of Surgeons.

The Royal Hospital provided a particular challenge for Cheselden, for it gave him unique scope to practice both his anatomical and surgical skills in an environment which he would not easily have found at St Thomas's, where he had spent twenty years, or at any of the other teaching hospitals. But more importantly, it gave him the opportunity to develop his administrative talents, rare in physicians and rarer still in surgeons. During his time at Chelsea he reorganized the surgical wards in the Infirmary, appointed a qualified nursing staff and cut down the cost of prescriptions which had reached astronomical proportions.* Above all, he was a kindly man, pre-occupied with the problem of pain and deeply concerned in the old soldiers committed to his charge. We do not know what those old soldiers felt about him, but although at his death he was not accorded a military funeral, thirty In-Pensioners followed his coffin to the grave in the Hospital Burial Ground.

William Cheselden's colleague for ten years at Chelsea was renowned less for his medical expertise than for his eccentricity. Dr Messenger Monsey was appointed Physician in 1742 and died a little short of his ninety-sixth birthday after forty-six colourful years at the Royal Hospital. He was an authentic eighteenth-century character, a man who made a virtue of bad manners, affected a studied disorder in his dress, and – like Robert Walpole – 'talked bawdy'. This, if it shocked his contemporaries, must have endeared him to the In-Pensioners, and his Infirmary rounds must have been redoubtable occasions.

Yet, despite his defects, his honesty and directness commended him to a wide and varied circle of friends. Chesterfield found him 'a monster of good humour'; Pope, Hogarth and Garrick were his constant companions; even the fastidious Horace Walpole dined out on his anecdotes. Johnson, almost alone of his contemporaries, disliked his crudeness, although more probably he envied his popularity. Boswell, who sat next to him at a Festival Dinner at Chelsea when the old man was nearly ninety, enjoyed his conversation and recorded his comment that 'Brandy was very pernicious for the Stomack'. Since eight different forms of alcohol were served on that occasion and the worthy physician indulged in all of them, he seems to have preached less honestly than he practised. He was a man for all seasons, if not for all tastes, and he died as he had lived, eccentric to the last, bequeathing his velvet coat to one friend and the buttons to another.

Many attempts were made during Dr Monsey's long tenure of office to appoint another physician in his place, but he developed a variety of wicked stratagems which effectively frightened off each competitor in turn. When finally he met his match and died in 1788,

* Between 1700 and 1735 the annual cost had risen from £300 to over £2,000.

he was succeeded by a man as different from him as it was possible to be.

Benjamin Moseley had been a regimental physician and Surgeon-General in Jamaica before his appointment to Chelsea. He was an authority on tropical diseases and hydrophobia, and as prolific in print as he was sparing in good humour. He occupied his position for thirty-one years during which time he presided over the building and equipping of Sir John Soane's new Infirmary on the site of Walpole House; and along the way he acquired – not without justification – a massive chip on his shoulder.

In 1801 or 1802, the Hospital Surgeon, Thomas Keate, had been granted a salary increase from £100 to £1,000 a year, which was twice what the Governor was receiving and nearly three times more than any other member of the Hospital staff. There is no recorded explanation for this sensational rise and we must assume that Keate had demanded the going rate then being earned by surgeons in civilian practice.

Dr Moseley, who was in theory Keate's superior, was left languishing on an annual salary of £100. This injury both to his pride and his pocket he bore with exemplary fortitude until in the summer of 1806 he steeled himself to address a long memorial to the Chelsea Board. In this mournful document he drew the Board's attention to the humiliating disparity between his own emoluments and those of the Surgeon. He goes on:

'I further understand that the Apothecary enjoys from £600 to £800 a year [*this was untrue*], who also has the advantage with regard to an apartment – and a very material one – as regards myself who has no such advantage [*he had elected to live in his own house at Fulham*]. I further understand that the Physician of Greenwich Hospital enjoys about £800 a year and it is in consideration to enlarge that sum. I thereby humbly solicit an increase.'

Confronted with these figures, the Board could scarcely resist Dr Moseley's request, but their decision – to increase his salary to £300 – was tantamount to a slap in the face. A year later they added injury to insult by increasing it further to £365. It was the last rise the unfortunate Physician received.

Yet despite their foibles – and their grievances – the medical officers of the Royal Hospital during the latter half of the eighteenth century were a devoted and dedicated band of men, and among them we should not forget the lady-killing Robert Adair ('Robin Adair' of popular memory), and the brilliant physician Dr Tessier.

The same could not be said of the eighteenth century Governors of the Hospital who, with two exceptions, were dull, disinterested, and usually devious. But the two distinguished soldiers who between them presided over the In-Pensioners from 1740 to 1795 were – in their very different ways – remarkable men. Under them the Pensioners prospered as never before – and as they were not to prosper again for over 100 years.

Lt. Gen. Sir Robert Rich was appointed in 1740. Wounded at Blenheim, his portrait, which hangs in the corridor of the Secretary's Office, shows him with a quizzical expression and a pirate's patch over one eye. In 1715, he had raised the 4th Regiment of Dragoons (eight of the first ten governors of the Royal Hospital were cavalry-men) and three years after his appointment to Chelsea he had led his regiment at the battle of Dettingen. On that occasion two In-Pensioners had followed their old Colonel overseas and to one of them, Sergeant Hinton, Sir Robert presented a snuff-box as a memento of this unusual regimental reunion. Fourteen years later, Rich was promoted to Field-Marshal, one of the first officers to hold that newly instituted rank.

Sir Robert's reign at Chelsea lasted for twenty-eight years. Like most of the Governors of the period, he continued to live at his private house in Grosvenor Square, while letting his official apartments at Chelsea to a succession of well-heeled tenants; and there is little doubt that he made a private fortune out of his public duties. The fact that he was also a member of Parliament must have helped.

His period of office is notable for the fact that he rarely, if ever, attended Board meetings. Instead, he communicated with the Hospital staff through the medium of written directives which descended upon his unfortunate subordinates in a steady stream. These orders show him to have been as eccentric as he was industrious. One of his first decisions was to appropriate the Officers' Hall and to move the Governor's Table there, much to the annoyance of the 'Captains' and Light Horsemen who found themselves obliged to take their meals with the other In-Pensioners. Why he should have done this is obscure, since he only dined with his staff on festive occasions.

Discipline was his particular hobby horse. Here is an order dated February 8, 1759:

> 'The Governor directs that one of the Sergeants of each Ward call over the Men belonging to that Ward each night a 9 o'clock and take care to turn out all Women and other Persons that have no Business there. In case of any resistance (sic!) he is to call the Guard to his assistance. If any men are missing or any Disturbance caused, he is to acquaint the Adjutant next morning.'

It seems to have had little effect, for fifty years later the then Governor, Sir David Dundas, delivered himself of the following broadside:

> 'The Governor cannot help expressing his Astonishment that in breach of Standing Orders it appears that 10 Women *have taken up Quarters* in the Wards of the Hospital. And that with two exceptions, the Persons who have so grossly violated these orders are all non-commissioned officers, who seem to forget that every Private Man in the House is as well entitled as they are to assume the liberty they have presumed to take. Two days will be allowed for the Women in question to provide themselves with Lodgings.'

Sir Robert's other obsession was dogs; and on August 23, 1760, he directed thus:

> 'The contagious distemper that at present rages too generally among Doggs in London & Westminster occasions His Excellency Sir Robert Rich to issue the following Orders, in hopes of preventing the like infection from reaching to Chelsea College:
> 'That every person whatever belonging to the College who has a Dogg or Doggs immediately take proper care that the same be tied up for the space of Six weeks from the date hereof. Any mad Dogg shall be destroyed by the Sentrys.'

At this date, there were no fewer than sixty-two dogs permanently installed in the Royal Hospital and the Governor's edict must have resulted in memorable chaos.

For much of Sir Robert Rich's Governorship the Pay Office was occupied by two men whose respective contributions to the Royal Hospital were very different indeed.

William Pitt became Paymaster in 1746. He inherited a situation where, as we have seen, the administration of out-pensions had become the subject of gross irregularities, unchecked in Walpole's time and greatly compounded since then, for by the middle of the century the number of Out-Pensioners had grown to nearly 10,000 with the reduction of the army after the Peace of Aix-la-Chapelle. The root cause of these evils lay in the system of deferring first payment of pensions for twelve months after admission to the list. Once in the clutches of the moneylenders, the old soldiers were sitting ducks and they were duly plucked and trussed in their hundreds.

Pitt, who conscientiously attended the meetings of the Chelsea Board, must have had a shrewd idea what was going on, but it was not until 1754 that he devised a remedy to these abuses. Tobias Smollett described it thus:

'(In this year) Mr Pitt brought in a bill which will ever remain a standing monument of his humanity. The poor disabled veterans who enjoyed the pension of Chelsea Hospital were so iniquitously oppressed by a set of miscreants . . . that many of them, with their families, were in danger of starving . . .

'Mr Pitt, perceiving that this evil originally flowed from the delay of the first payment . . ., removed the necessity of borrowing by providing that a half year's pension should be advanced half year *before* it is due . . . and that all contracts should be void by which any pension might be mortgaged . . .'

It seemed too good to be true; and it was. Although the Out-Pensioners now got their money in advance, it reached them only after a deduction of 1s. in the pound to meet the inflated interest charges on what was, in effect, a loan. It was a classic Irishman's rise.

Pitt's successor as Paymaster-General was Henry Fox, later Lord Holland, the younger son of Sir Stephen Fox by his second marriage. During the eight years of his period of office the conduct of affairs at the Hospital reached a new low level. Virtually every position from the Adjutant to the sculleryman was filled by nominees of Fox's political friends – so much so that an anonymous biographer of old Dr Monsey observed: 'The College at Chelsea, which ought to have been devoted to national charity, was over-run by valets, grooms or election-jobbers. . . . By this preposterous misapplication of public rewards, a man, by shaving the Paymaster, brushing his coat . . . or marrying his mistress, became the companion of a General, a Physician and a Divine.' Henry Fox himself followed the practice of all his predecessors, save only the honest Pitt, by appropriating the

147

interest on large balances of money voted for the Army. Thus were the fortunes of the House of Holland secured.

As usual, the pensioners were left to fend for themselves, as this sad little story from the Board Minutes shows:

> 'Hugh Brown of Capt d'Arboledo's Independent Company at Jersey submits a petition representing that after 35 years Service in Sir Bevill Greenville's Regt. he was ordered to be taken into the said Company in which he has served 25 years and being now discharged from thence after *sixty years service* in the Army and 87 years of age, prays to have the benefit of the Out-Pension.'

Shamefacedly the Board agreed and back-dated the award two years. Hugh Brown had waited a long time for his 5*d*. a day.

In 1768, Lt. Gen. Sir George Howard was appointed Governor. Like his predecessor he lived in Grosvenor Square and was a member of Parliament; but there the similarity ended, for General Howard was a wise and kindly man and one of the great servants of the Royal Hospital. His portrait also hangs in the corridor of the Secretary's Office, a handsome old gentleman with the air of a family solicitor and a touch of the benevolent martinet. Under his guidance the Hospital enjoyed its first unbroken period of calm, free of scandal and innocent of those criminal practices from which the name of Chelsea had become inseparable.

George Howard had been commissioned into the army at the age of eight and had commanded the Buffs at Fontenoy and Culloden. Subsequently, he became Colonel of the 1st Dragoon Guards and, like Sir Robert Rich, was promoted to Field-Marshal. More than any other previous Governor, he devoted himself to the happiness and well-being of the In-Pensioners, and the archives are full of small but revealing examples of his constant care for his old soldiers. Even when he bristled, it was usually with good reason:

> 'The Governor positively orders that no man of what station so ever in the Wards carry lighted candles into his Chamber for fear of setting fire to it. Pensioners are not to take the candles out of the lanthorns which are provided for their benefit and safety.'

When necessary, he could both bark and bite:

> 'Whereas the shamefull Practice of selling provisions is a most

wicked prostitution of this Noble Charity, instituted for the
happiness and comfort of Deserving and Meritorious old Soldiers,
and whereas the Standing order against such Shamefull Practice
has been disobeyed by many: The Governor this day [*December 10,
1780*] saw a flagrant instance of it in Robert Goulder of the 11th
Ward who in open defiance of the said order sold his provisions to
a Woman in the Piazza, for which he is ordered to be turned out
of the House.'

But always he was compassionate:

'The Governor desires that action be taken to appoint Pensioners to take food to those in the Wards who are too infirm to
help themselves and who have grown grey together in the Service
of their King and Country. There is no knowing when each of us
may find himself in the same need of comfort and understanding.'

This good and dedicated man was to enjoy – too briefly, as it
proved – the support of a Paymaster cast in the same mould, in the
person of Edmund Burke.

Burke first went to the Pay Office in April 1782 and stayed six
months. He returned again in 1783 for a further year. His most
lasting memorial was his Pay Office Act, which, among many other
wise reforms, brought to an end the system of poundage deductions
from army pay.* Up to this date some £5,000,000 had been withheld
from soldiers' pay but less than half this amount had been spent on
the Royal Hospital. The rest had vanished in out-pensions, Exchequer fees and a century of fraudulent conversion. Now at least
Burke had put Hospital funds beyond the reach of itching fingers,
and his own sense of financial rectitude was underlined by the
economies he effected at the Pay Office, not least in respect of his
own salary.

As we look back at the eighteenth century the figure of Edmund
Burke stands head and shoulders above most of his contemporaries –
a tireless champion of social justice and civil liberty. He was, in
Churchill's phrase 'perhaps the greatest man that Ireland has produced'. He was devoted to the Royal Hospital and was a constant
visitor, talking to the old soldiers and walking through the wards
(something no *Paymaster* had done before him). His kindness and
compassion are illustrated in a Board Minute of August 1, 1783.

* Poundage continued to be deducted from the pay of Household troops
until 1831. The deduction of 1s. in the pound from out-pensions continued
until 1847, although reduced to 6d. by Lord John Russell in his reforms of 1833.

A Captain Pemble of Fort George had written to the Commissioners regarding men discharged from his Invalid Company. 'I cannot,' he says, 'help expressing my Pity for poor old men who have compleated their Service and will be obliged to undertake a round Journey of 1100 miles to and from London when many of them will probably finish their Journey on the Road.'

The Secretary was instructed to reply to Capt. Pemble and acquaint him that the Board had no legal power to dispense with the appearance of these men. In his own hand, Edmund Burke added this comment in the margin: 'This is a harsh and needless imposition. If such is the Law, then it is time in all conscience that the Law were changed.'

Sir George Howard was not only a great Governor. He was also a hospitable one, and during his period of office the Hospital became renowned as a centre for entertainment. This took the form of musical evenings in the Great Hall and the Chapel which the In-Pensioners were permitted to attend; and, for a more exclusive circle, the annual Festival Dinners held on Founder's Day and the King's Birthday.

These Festival Dinners were elaborate affairs, starting at 11 a.m., and continuing, through seven or eight courses and a formidable assortment of liquor, until three o'clock in the afternoon. They were held in the former Officers' Hall (now the In-Pensioners' billiard room) and the seating-plan at the two tables illustrates the niceties of the Royal Hospital pecking-order.

At the head of the first table sat the Governor with fifteen senior members of his staff to whom was added, upon his appointment as organist in 1783, the celebrated Dr Charles Burney. Over the second table presided the Surgeon's Mate and below him sat the junior servants, including the Keeper of the Lights, the gardener and even the sculleryman. The Surgeon's Mate was required not only to keep strict order among his curiously assorted flock but also to minister discreetly to anyone who might be overcome by the Governor's generous hospitality.

Invitations to the Festival Dinners were highly prized and the most regular attendant for many years was James Boswell. He was present for the first time on Founder's Day, 1783 as the guest of Edmund Burke and seems to have greatly commended himself to

General Howard who forthwith gave him a standing invitation to all subsequent dinners. Unfortunately the guest lists have not survived, but from Boswell's journal it is clear that General Howard's taste was catholic and he enjoyed the company of intelligent and even eccentric men from many walks of life. At his first dinner, Boswell found himself sitting between his host, Edmund Burke, and Dr Monsey, who delighted his literary companion by keeping up a flow of bawdy anecdotes throughout the meal. On a subsequent occasion he sat next to Charles Burney who was to occupy the post of organist at the Hospital for thirty-one years and completed his great *History of Music* in his second-floor apartment overlooking Light Horse Court.

Boswell has left this record of his last Festival Dinner in 1790:

> 'It was an excellent dinner, as usual, and I drank of all the liquors: cold drink, small beer, ale, porter, cyder, madeira, sherry, old hock, port, Claret. I was in good spirits at the festival, talked well, and was pleased, as the table began to thin, to find Mr Keate [*the Surgeon*] come and sit by me and carry on some intelligent conversation.
>
> 'I drank a glass of cherry brandy at Dawson's, and went to town in Trapaud's coach . . .
>
> 'I was much intoxicated, and I suppose talked nonsense . . . Very irregular this; but I thought the festival an excuse.'

They say the eighteenth century was the Age of Reason. It also seems to have been the Age of Stamina.

With the appointment of the austere and unsociable General Sir David Dundas in 1804, the Festival Dinners were reduced to purely domestic functions* at which the guests were strictly limited both in number and intellectual accomplishment. The new Governor's intentions were set out in a long Garrison Order, no less, which directed the cooks to provide a meal of three courses 'without going to expensive and unseasonable Niceties'. There was still a generous selection of drinks although claret and madeira were served only at the first table and not to the junior staff. Boswell would not have enjoyed himself.

While the *haut-monde* came and went upon their social occasions at Chelsea, the other, more humble world of the In-Pensioners trod

---

* The Governor's Table, as such, had been abolished in 1796.

its different, primrose path. By the middle of the eighteenth century, the Hospital was no longer isolated in a rural landscape. It still retained its village atmosphere, but the old soldiers could now find their local entertainments without travelling far afield. The Bun House in Pimlico Road was probably a little tame for their taste and a little pricey for their pockets, but the growing traffic of Out-Pensioners attending upon the Secretary's Office for their money had resulted in a flurry of new ale-houses, and an enterprising publican had opened the Royal Hospital Tavern opposite the London Gate, within staggering distance of the Main Guardhouse.

The spread of newspapers during this period has given us some sidelights on the tiny dramas of daily life in and around the Hospital. Here are a few cameos:

'A lamentable tragedy occurred last Thursday when a boat overturned opposite Chelsea Steps drowning all save an old Pentioner out of Chelsea College who swam ashore and was rescued.' (1753)

'A Chelsea Pensioner sat in the stocks at St Ann's, Soho, for the space of one Hour, for prophane cursing and swearing.' (1755)

'On Sunday last a Chelsea Pensioner saved from drowning a small child that had fallen into the Westbourne stream. For his good behaving, he was given one shilling by the Parish.' (1759)

About the same time, the *Gentleman's Magazine* carried a letter from a country squire who had recently paid his first visit to the Hospital. He was duly impressed by the peace and dignity of Wren's buildings although disenchanted with Gibbons' statue of 'the effeminate Charles, who had never figured in any wars but those of Venus, crowned with laurels.' He then goes on:

'Presently I approached an old veteran on the Piazza [*the Colonnade*] with empty sleeve and care-worn face, and engaged him in conversation.

'"Have you been long in the College?" I asked.

'"Eight years, your Honour."

'"I have noticed that there are some who do not, like you, bear the marks of age or wounds. Are there many such?"

'He replied, a little melancholy;

'"A Friend at Court is of more essential service to a man than a body covered with scars and wounds. Tho' my mother bore me on the field of battle and my whole life has been devoted to military services, I should never have obtained a retreat here had I not had a *more powerful* recommendation."

'We were standing near the Great Porch and my new acquaintance invited me to view the hall where the veterans are entertained, and also the Chapell. I was much moved by the simple dignity of these places where the very stones are full of history.

'As I took my leave, I offered him coin, but he uncovered and bowed in very gentlemanly fashion. "Your pleasure is my reward, Sir," he said, and I went away marvelling greatly.'

This charming story tells us two things. First, it seems that patronage applied not only to offices of profit at the Royal Hospital but even to the right of admission for ordinary soldiers; and secondly, that courtesy has always been the badge of nature's gentlemen.

On May 6, 1779, the Royal Hospital broke new ground with the first performance at the Theatre Royal, Covent Garden of Charles Dibdin's comic opera *The Chelsea Pensioner*. It ran for four nights and then sank without trace. Nonetheless Dibdin's plot has diverting possibilities.

The chief character is an old veteran of Marlborough's wars with the unoriginal name of Blenheim. His Pensioner friends are Malplaquet, Plunder, Thicket, Flint and Birch. Blenheim's daughter, Nancy, is hotly pursued by the Governor's son, Lively, much to the indignation of Lapstone, the villainous Adjutant, who has designs on her himself. Lapstone's efforts to frame Blenheim are thwarted by his old comrades and the opera ends with the Adjutant being fired and the Governor promoting Blenheim to sergeant. Nancy and Lively are joined in happy matrimony.

The music is tuneful but unremarkable and includes a love-duet; a patter song by Plunder about the parlous condition of Pensioners; and – what else, indeed! – two rollicking drinking choruses. A revival in the Great Hall with a Royal Hospital cast would be a riot.

'Donald Macleod,' runs another news item, 'a former In-Pensioner of His Majesty's Royal Hospital at Chelsea, and 101 years of age, has recently walked from Inverness to London. His second wife, who has a son aged 6, is shortly to be delivered of another child, and the soldier Macleod seeks therefore to have an increase of his pension.' (1789)

A few years earlier, the In-Pensioners had joined the hustings. During the election campaign of 1783, Sir Cecil Wray, one of the candidates, had proposed the closing down of the Royal Hospital as an economy measure. Up spoke the old gentlemen with the following petition:

> 'It having been reported to us by two of our Sarjiants and some other of our Corps that can read that your Honour has come to a Resolution to demolish our Hospital, and send us poor crippled and aged souls helpless into the world again, we were drawn out on our parade yesterday, and came to the Resolution of calling upon your Worship and to state to you —
> 'That as we are all old Soldiers, and like to talk about nothing but battles, and how we lost our precious limbs, and what we did, and all that, we would not value life at a cartridge box if we could not see one another and compare old squares . . .
> 'That if your Honour goes on there can be no other way for us but to ax relief from all good Christians in the streets, and to pray God to help us, which to be sure will be damn'd hard after all our sufferings.
> 'Hoping that as your Honour is partly a Soldier and may sometime or other see sarvice yourself, Your Honour wont take the bread out of our mouths, but leave us a house and belly-full for our shattered carcases at sixty. And as in duty bound we shall ever pray for your Worship.'

This splendid exercise in Churchillian impudence was signed by three sergeants, two corporals and one private, with 761 'marks', which was 300 more than the number of In-Pensioners in the Royal Hospital.

On October 7, 1801, the *Morning Chronicle* reported the only recorded case of murder at the Royal Hospital.

It appeared that a protracted argument had raged between two In-Pensioners – a 'Captain' and a Private – over the allocation of coal for burning in their Ward. The quarrel was patched up by the Major, but some months later open warfare was declared again. The report continues:

> 'On the morning of the day when the fatal catastrophe took place, the prisoner entering the room of the deceased said "you must get up and fight me", accompanying his words by holding out a pistol. The deceased without making any reply contented himself with knocking the pistol out of his hand. The prisoner immediately discharged another pistol, the contents of which pierced the heart of the deceased, who instantly expired. On examining the pistol offered to the deceased, it appeared that it only contained a ball without any powder.'

The prisoner was duly found guilty and executed, maintaining to the last that he had not offered the deceased an unloaded firearm.

In these and many other ways, the In-Pensioners had now acquired fame – and notoriety. Emerging from their monastic retreat, they had become part of the London scene, quaintly-dressed survivals from another age, but far from quaint in their appetite for life. They had been lucky to survive the last century. They were going to need even more luck to survive the next.

10

From Waterloo to Mons

It is a hundred years from Waterloo to Mons, and only 30 miles on the map. Between them they mark the high noon of Empire and the summit of British influence and achievement. Yet in this century of profound change lie buried also the seeds of future decay.

We pick up our story in 1806, a few years before Wellington's famous victory. In that year William Windham introduced his Pensions Act which ended a century of parsimony and injustice and created the basis from which our modern system of Army pensions has developed.

The effect of Windham's Act was to make all pensions a matter of legal *right* instead of a bounty proceeding from the Crown. Men who previously could not have received more than 5d. a day could now *demand* as much as 2s., dependent on length of service, climate in which that service had been performed,* nature of wounds, and degree of disability. These changes had a dramatic effect. At the end of 1806, there were 21,177 Out-Pensioners at an annual cost of £180,263 19s. 3½d. In 1807, after the introduction of the Act, the number of Out-Pensioners fell slightly to 20,805 at a cost of £357,222 7s. 3½d. – almost exactly double the previous year. The Out-Pensioners were delighted. The Army hierarchy was dis-enchanted.

The In-Pensioners, who had of course surrendered their pensions on admission to the Hospital, were quick to sniff an advantage and the Board was soon confronted with a flood of requests to revert to out-pension at the new and much more attractive rates. But the Governor, Sir David Dundas, would have none of that. On October 7, 1807 he issued an instruction to the effect that any In-Pensioner wishing to revert would do so at his *old*, pre-Windham rate, and then only at the Governor's discretion. It was at least arguable that he had no authority for such a decision, but as Governor he was in a fair position to make his own rules.

---

* For example, two years in India or the West Indies counted for three years ordinary service. This distinction was short-lived and was abolished in 1818.

The revolutionary principle behind Windham's Act did not long survive the military prejudices of the day. It was repealed in 1826 on the pretext that its working was prejudicial to good order and military discipline since it provided commanding officers with a simple excuse for prematurely discharging 'unsatisfactory' soldiers. Thus, in the words of Lord Hardinge, 'good men were compelled to remain in their corps, and the bad had the advantage of being early pensioned for life.' With the repeal of the Act, soldiers ceased to have a legal *right* to a pension, although the new and more generous rates remained in force. The startling impact of the end of the Napoleonic wars and the administrative transfer of Kilmainham out-pensions to Chelsea is shown in these figures, covering the twenty years between the passing of the Act and its repeal:

	Out-Pensioners	*Cost*
1807	20,805	£ 357,222
1826	82,734	£1,381,128

General Sir David Dundas had been appointed Governor of the Royal Hospital in 1804. A soldier of no great distinction, he was the nominee of the Commander-in-Chief, the Duke of York, whom he briefly succeeded in that office in 1809, combining his duties at the War Office with those at Chelsea.

He was a dry, aloof puritan and he ruled the Royal Hospital with an excess of regimental zeal. At least he was no absentee landlord for he was the first Governor for nearly a century to occupy his official apartments, and this was bad luck on the In-Pensioners, as the following Garrison Order of November 30, 1804, shows:

'The practice which has gradually crept into the Garrison of keeping Poultry has increased to such a degree as to have become a common nuisance particularly to the Sick who from the Break of Day are disturbed with the crowing of Cocks and cackling of Hens ... which are otherwise Pernicious and Disagreeable. The Governor having noted the Unmilitary Appearance of the Flank Square which more resembles a Farm than a Barrack is pleased to order that this Practice will cease. He is further pleased to order that the keeping of Dogs in the Wards will cease [*yes, they were still there*].'

This effectively deprived the In-Pensioners of one profitable side-line. General Dundas now trained his guns on another:

'Serjt Alexander Smith of the 16th Ward having been convicted of the enormous crime of making away not only with his own necessaries, but with 2 Hatts, 2 Great Coats, 2 Uniform Coats, 2 Waistcoats, 2 pair of Breaches, 2 prs of Shoes, and 4 pair of Stockings, the Governor, General Sir David Dundas, is pleased to order that the said Serjeant Alexander Smith be disgracefully turned out of the House without a Pension. The noncommissioned officers are in future to prevent the admission of Jews and old-cloths men into their respective Wards. . . .'

The Governor showed no mercy either to dishonest servants of the Hospital. On May 8, 1806, the Master Cook, James Morris died suddenly. A week later, William Bramley, the second cook, was dismissed for purloining large quantities of oatmeal and salt supplied for making the pensioners' broth, and his sentence was promulgated in Garrison Orders 'to deter others from committing any such nefarious abuses in future.'

Bramley then delivered himself of a lachrymose appeal to the Commissioners:

'My Lords, may I presume to implore your reconsideration of that most awful sentence you were pleased to pass upon me! Mr Morris being dead is unable to be spoke with on my behalf.

'Oh, that I could convey to you the feelings of an afflicted Father with a most unfortunate and distressed Family, continually bewailling themselves with all the apprehensions of woe and want. Oh, affliction upon affliction! Oh, woe! Death itself would have been preferable to me rather than have suffered what I have done. I pray that mercy may induce you to change that awful sentence into forgiveness and reinstate me.'

Then, as an afterthought:

'If that is not to be, Oh, my Lords, may I be admitted to hope, may I *dare* to solicit some compensation for my past services?'

William Bramley was out of luck. Among the effects of the late James Morris was found an unposted letter to the Board setting forth the many and detailed malpractices of William Bramley. He stayed sacked – and uncompensated.

❧

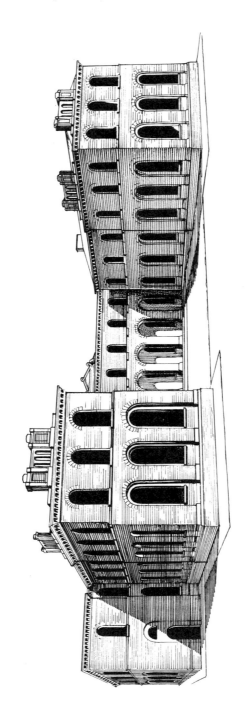

Sir John Soane's Infirmary, opened in 1816 and destroyed by enemy action in 1941

The most significant event of Sir David Dundas's Governorship was the building of the new Infirmary. The increase in the number of Out-Pensioners during the eighteenth century had resulted in a growing demand for admission to the Royal Hospital, and simultaneously the Napoleonic wars had put an increasing pressure on the limited resources of Wren's old Infirmary. Various temporary expedients had failed to solve these problems and by 1806 the situation had become critical.

In February General Dundas proposed that the Board should acquire the lease of Walpole House to preserve the Hospital's western boundary and that Ranelagh Gardens, derelict for the past three years, should be purchased as the site either of a new military hospital or an extension to house an additional 300 In-Pensioners. The Treasury refused to sanction either proposal on the grounds of cost, whereupon the Ranelagh Estate was bought by a General Wilford and the grounds of Walpole House were leased, quite improperly, to Lt. Col. Gordon, the Duke of York's Secretary.* Both these developments were to cost the Royal Hospital dear.

At this point Benjamin Moseley, the Physician, suggested the acquisition and conversion of Walpole House as a new Infirmary, thus releasing Wren's old building in Infirmary Court as accommodation for additional In-Pensioners. His proposal was hotly contested on a number of valid grounds by the new Clerk of the Works, John Soane, but the intransigence of the Treasury – and the Board's indecision – had left no alternative; and in 1809 work began. In the event, the conversion of Walpole House involved its complete reconstruction and, more seriously, the demolition of nearly all Wren's elegant buildings on the west side of Infirmary Court.† When the work was completed in 1816, the new Infirmary provided beds for eighty patients and accommodation for the nursing staff while the space made available in Infirmary Court and the old Infirmary annexe in the East wing housed sixty-three additional In-Pensioners, raising the establishment to 539. Some fifty years later, an extension to the Infirmary provided beds for a further twenty-one patients and the Hospital establishment was increased to its maximum total of 558.

Soane's Infirmary survived for 125 years until, on April 16, 1941

* Here he proceeded to build Gordon House, designed by Thomas Leverton and still in use today as Officers' Quarters.

† They were subsequently replaced by the featureless buildings which stand there today, designed by Soane regardless of style or harmonization and constructed in a tasteless yellow brick.

it was destroyed by a land-mine, with numerous casualties. It had never been a particularly happy inspiration.

Col. Gordon's intrusion upon Royal Hospital property was significant in one particular respect. It was to prove the last occasion on which the Hospital was exposed to those abuses and corrupt practices which had bedevilled it since the day it was founded. Henceforth its management and administration – not least on the financial side – were to be conducted with exemplary propriety. While this resulted in good husbandry, it made for colourless characters, and the history of the next hundred years is marked by a succession of worthy but unremarkable Governors and administrators. There were, however, two notable exceptions.

Lord John Russell was appointed Paymaster-General in 1830 and was to hold that office for four years. This 'marvellous little man', as Charles Greville described him, soon brought his reforming zeal to Chelsea. He had at first inclined to the belief that the Hospital was an unnecessary institution, but a closer acquaintance with the In-Pensioners converted him into a convinced advocate of King Charles's 'noble charity'.

1833 was Russell's *annus mirabilis* and we may here summarize his varied activity during that year.

The poundage on out-pensions was reduced from 1*s*. to 6*d*., payment was made quarterly in advance, and In-Pensioners were paid weekly.

The establishment of the Royal Hospital was ruthlessly pruned and fourteen staff appointments were abolished while eight others were merged into four new offices. The In-Pensioners were reorganized into six companies under newly-appointed officers 'of long standing in the army or who have been disabled', under the title of Captains of Invalids, 'with largely nominal duties'.

Allotment gardens were provided for In-Pensioners and recreation facilities in the Great Hall, which was closed for communal messing and meals were supplied to the old soldiers in their wards (a decision which Russell may well have regretted later).

Daily services in the Chapel were discontinued and the post of Second Chaplain abolished, while six In-Pensioners were trained as choristers.

The former regulations of 1703 were revived and strictly enforced with the result that all appointments at the Hospital, other than that of Clerk of the Works, were reserved for retired officers and soldiers, and the practice of patronage was severely frowned upon, although never entirely eradicated.

Finally the officers of the House were given permission by William IV to wear 'Windsor uniform', a dress designed by George III and still worn on formal occasions at the Hospital, although much altered and adapted to suit modern requirements. Similarly, the In-Pensioners' uniforms, scarcely changed since Marlborough's day, were re-designed and, as we have seen, progressively adopted from 1841 onwards.

While this silent revolution was taking place, the daily management of the Hospital proceeded under Russell's able chairmanship. Around this period, the Chelsea Board seems to have been more than usually involved in the misdemeanours of Out-Pensioners. While the Commissioners were in no way concerned with the administration of justice, each case was referred to them where the continuance of a man's pension might be in question. Sometimes – although not often – they showed a delicate sense of tact.

The Chief Constable of the Irish village of Mountmellick reported that on July 18, 1833 James Murphy, a pensioner from the 5th Foot at 9d. a day who had lost an arm at Waterloo, 'behaved himself in an exceedingly improper manner by getting intoxicated, calling the police force "Parish-fed Bastards, Orange [*here follows a most eloquent blank space*], and Brunswickers", and by going in front of the houses of the Clerk of the Church and Postmaster and giving them gross abuse in terms of uncouth obscenity.' The full majesty of the Irish law proceeds: 'By so doing he succeeded in inflaming the passions of this once troubled but now tranquil locality. It is very likely that his conduct will have the most undesirable political consequences.'

Russell and his colleagues contemplated this fearful warning of impending insurrection with praiseworthy calm and – tongue in cheek – duly delivered a Solomon's judgement – thus. 'Intoxication is a vice not unknown among old soldiers. It is an endemic disease among old Irish soldiers. Politics is a pastime among Englishmen. It is a passion among Irishmen. Neither passion nor disease are subjects for their Lordships' discrimination, but as a mark of their displeasure they are pleased to reduce this man's pension by 1d. a day.' History does not record what further uncouth obscenities passed the lips of James Murphy when this intelligence reached him.

The Russell reforms had largely concentrated on domestic issues at the Royal Hospital. Now the net was to be cast wider. In 1846, Russell succeeded Sir Robert Peel as Prime Minister. The office of Paymaster-General in the new administration went to Thomas Macaulay who had declined a more influential portfolio so that he might have time to pursue his literary interests. Macaulay's two years at the Pay Office were marked by a compassion and understanding unusual among politicians of the mid-nineteenth century. He was regular in his attendance at meetings of the Chelsea Board and a Minute of February, 1847 is very much in character. The Board had approved the award of pensions to long-service soldiers of West Indian regiments and throughout the Minute these men are referred to as 'Negro soldiers'. In each such reference Macaulay has crossed out the word 'Negro' and inserted in his own hand the word 'Black'.

His logical – and prudent – mind is also reflected in the decision to discontinue the system of multiple victualling contractors (historically the cause of endless trouble), and on March 9 John Gillett of Silver Street, Bloomsbury was appointed sole supplier to the Hospital of 'the whole ration of provisions – viz. Beef, Mutton, Bread, Cheese, Salt, Oatmeal, Cocoa and Sugar at 9¼d. per head per day.'

But the decision of lasting importance was the introduction of an Act in October, 1847 by which the poundage deductions from out-pensions were finally ended and the cost of out-pensions and the entire maintenance of the Royal Hospital were henceforth met out of Parliamentary Votes.* By this Act the country surrendered about £50,000 a year in favour of the Out-Pensioners who for the first time in 162 years now received their pensions in full. It was the logical extension of Russell's reform of 1833 and he was undoubtedly the moving spirit behind Macaulay's Act.

The Royal Hospital's revenue was now confined to three sources: the Army Prize Fund, legacies, and rents received from Hospital property.†

The Army Prize Fund had its origin in Lord Palmerston's Act of 1811, whereby the distribution of unclaimed sums of money remaining in the hands of untrustworthy prize agents was brought under Parliamentary control. Under the Act the Chelsea Board were

* From 1681 to 1847, the Army contributed to the Royal Hospital revenue from all sources £8,132,921 9s. 10¼d.

† It is still known as the 'Prize and Legacy Fund' and is administered at the sole discretion of the Commissioners.

appointed recipients of all such sums and any monies unclaimed after a specified period were to be applied to the general purposes of the Hospital. The subsequent Army Prize Act of 1832 vested in the Commissioners the responsibility for the distribution of prize monies direct to claimants. Some indication of the amount involved may be gathered from the Chelsea accounts which show a net income in the Hospital's favour of £590,000 between the passing of the 1811 Act and the year 1847. Had this fund been allowed to mature over the years, the Hospital would have been self-financing in perpetuity, but the long arm of the Treasury clawed back over half a million pounds in aid of Parliamentary Votes – and once again Chelsea Peter was robbed to pay Westminster Paul.

The most significant of the Royal Hospital legacies was that of Colonel John Drouly who in 1818 bequeathed the sum of £25,069 'to be applied for the use and benefit of the Pensioners in such manner as the Governors shall from time to time order and direct.' The 'Governors' at once proceeded to put a very liberal interpretation on Col. Drouly's intention by applying £20,970 of the bequest to purchasing back all but three acres of the Ranelagh Estate which had come on the market after the death of General Wilford. Nonetheless the Drouly Legacy has continued to serve the In-Pensioners generously and we will have occasion to refer to it again in a later chapter.

Thus, by the middle of the nineteenth century, important and far-reaching reforms had changed the face of the Royal Hospital. As always, the In-Pensioners were the beneficiaries of those few but dedicated men who had taken the trouble to read Charles II's Royal Warrant – and who, having read it, honoured it. In the whole history of Chelsea there are perhaps no more than twenty such men and to them the In-Pensioners owe an incalculable debt.

The years that followed the enlightened administration of men like Russell and Macaulay are largely overshadowed by the political and industrial conflicts of the day. In 1852, the Duke of Wellington had laid in state in the Great Hall and with his passing a whole Augustan age had ended. Four years later the same Great Hall was the scene of the farcical inquiry into the conduct of the Crimean War. The British Army – and particularly its whitewashed Generals – had become objects of public ridicule and contempt. The descent from

Olympus to the Styx had been sudden, headlong – and by no means unmerited.

By now the Royal Hospital had learned to expect no favours. It had become an oasis in a sea of public opprobrium, in a literal as well as a metaphorical sense.

In 1845, the decision to drive a main thoroughfare across Burton's Court had created the first breach in Christopher Wren's architectural defences. Now, in the 1850s, the construction of Chelsea Bridge Road and the building of the Embankment completed the triumph of vandalism over two centuries of taste. Within five years, Wren's South Terrace and his water garden were sacrificed to the demands of a new and hungry environment which swallowed elegance and converted it into expediency. In all London to-day there is no sadder sight than the desecrated South Grounds of the Royal Hospital.

And yet this indestructible village pursued the even tenor of its way. The Board Minutes of the year 1858, chosen at random, show that the pulse was still strong, the heartbeat firm, if occasionally erratic:

April 4.

'Joseph Taylor of the 95th Rifles, having lost an arm at Waterloo, is to be provided with an artificial limb of a new and revolutionary design.'

May 12.

'The Treasury recommend the transfer to the War Office of all business relating to the admission of Discharged Soldiers to the Pension List [*this is the first suggestion for transferring out-pension responsibility from Chelsea to Whitehall*].'

June 6.

'The Saint George's Club pray to be allowed the privilege of playing at Cricket upon one of the Plots of Land in front of the Hospital. – Answer: No.'

July 17.

'Tender for In-Pensioners greatcoats at 23*s.* 9*d.* each [*this compares with the cost of Ranelagh's 'surtout' coats at £1 in 1712*].'

July 20.

'Whitster's account for washing Hospital linen for the June quarter:

Articles washed:	37,436
Price:	£97–3–0d.'

October 9.

'Richard Rivers, late 14th Dragoons, to be dismissed the Hospital for misconduct and habitual Drunkenness. He is stated to be a great disturber of the comfort of the other Men in the Ward, disregarding the authority of non-commissioned officers, and consorting with disreputable Women in the Quadrangle.'

October 10.

'Award of contract for supplying the Clothing for the In-Pensioners to Favell & Bousfield of 12, St Mary Axe – the whole mounting to cost £3,039–4–11d.'

And on November 11 – prophetic date – the first Crimean veteran entered the Royal Hospital.

The repercussions of the Crimean War were soon followed by those of the Indian Mutiny; and in 1868, Edward Cardwell, Secretary of State for War in Gladstone's first administration, was appointed to investigate and report upon the whole steaming midden of Army organization and administration. His conclusions were fearless and damning. Astonishingly – despite diehard opposition – they were accepted and implemented almost in their entirety.

We need not concern outselves here with the full details of his report but the three most significant recommendations were these: the introduction of a system of limited engagement; the abolition of commission by purchase; the reorganization of infantry regiments on a two-battalion 'county' basis. From these proposals emerged, in embryo, the small, highly professional army which half a century later was to win immortality for itself on the same fields where Marlborough's soldiers, and Wellington's, had already shown the way.

The Cardwell reforms, and in particular the Short Service Act of 1870, had an immediate effect upon the out-pension establishment since they changed the entire basis of qualification and further introduced a number of innovations such as good conduct pay. The reforms were not directly concerned with the status of In-Pensioners at Chelsea and they would probably not have become involved but for the course of events in an unexpected quarter.

In 1865, an Act had been passed closing down the Royal Naval Hospital at Greenwich. The underlying reasons for this decision need not concern us here and are perhaps best left discreetly veiled, but over a period of years the number of naval In-Pensioners had been reduced from 2,710 to 1,400, when the Greenwich Hospital Act was passed. A few years earlier a Royal Commission had reported on the impact of the run-down:

'The practical effect of these reductions is at once offensive and demoralizing. They induce many pensioners to present themselves before visitors to this great national Asylum in the character of ordinary beggars; they force others to seek, in places of the lowest description about Greenwich, menial and degrading employments, and they tend to exclude the pensioners from social intercourse with all but those of their own monotonous fraternity; thereby' – the Report adds darkly – 'aggravating the evils which attend all monastic institutions.'

However, the old sailors were generously treated. Between 1865 and 1868, when Greenwich Hospital finally closed, all men reverting to outside status were paid 2s. a day in addition to their normal pensions and were further entitled to claim priority for admission, whether temporary or permanent, to any naval hospital.

It was not long before questions began to be raised about the Royal Hospital. If Greenwich was dispensable, how about Chelsea? If the arithmetic made sense with sailors, why not also with soldiers? And in March, 1870 Mr Gladstone set up a Committee under Capt. the Hon. J. C. Vivian, M.P. 'to inquire into the comparative advantages of in-door and out-door (sic) pensions for the numbers who can be accommodated at Chelsea.'

It at once became apparent that the two problems were very different, partly because of the recent history of Greenwich and partly because of the dissimilar attitudes of the services involved.

At the date of the inquiry there were 538 In-Pensioners at Chelsea and 64,000 Out-Pensioners (four times the naval figure), yet over the previous fifteen years the annual average of applications for admission to the Royal Hospital was only 172. The evidence indicated an almost total disinterest in the Hospital among serving and retired soldiers. It also threw up some interesting sidelights.

The committee's knowledge of the history of the Hospital in general and of army pensions in particular was shown to be both superficial and highly inaccurate; the net daily cost of maintaining each In-Pensioner was 2s. 3d., exactly the same as it had been 100 years before; the youngest In-Pensioner was 23 and the oldest 94; the Secretary, Major-General Hutt, and the Quartermaster both admitted that they had no direct contact of any kind with the In-Pensioners; and the examination of Sergeant-Major Lemuel George by a member of the Committee produced this brisk exchange:

'I believe there have been about seven dismissals a year? – About six or seven.

'What are the causes generally of the men being dismissed? – Habitual drunkenness, insubordination, or selling their clothing.

'What does the insubordination arise from? – From drink.'

The Committee took evidence from a large number of In-Pensioners and asked this question: 'If your out-pension rate were to be increased to 2*s.* a day, would you still wish to remain in the Hospital or would you prefer to revert?' Predictably there were as many different answers as there were men interviewed, and some of the replies were a little unexpected. For example:

John Barlow, late 24th Foot
Out-Pension rate 6d; is a native of Coventry; was at the Battle of Talavcra, and 'would like to be a Peeping Tom'; has had two wives and wants 'to be sent to Coventry to have another one.'

J. Mealy, late 77th Foot
Out-Pension rate 10*d.*; served in Crimea and India; would like to go out if he could get 2/– a day; never discusses these things in his ward; has heard of Greenwich but does not know what or where it is.

W. Hayes, late 4th Dragoons
Out-Pension rate 6*d.*; is very comfortable; has no friends either outside or in the Hospital; does not miss what he has not got.

The Committee duly reported that any saving produced by closing down the Royal Hospital would be so small as to have no material effect upon the out-pension rates of more than an insignificant number of men; and that any such saving would be more than offset by the cost of looking after the permanently crippled and infirm In-Pensioners in other establishments. After the fashion of all Committees, a number of recommendations were made, none of which were remotely practicable, and none of which were accordingly acted upon. In-Pensioner Barlow of Coventry was duly left to dream of Lady Godiva and an uneasy calm descended once again on the Royal Hospital.

Thirteen years later continuing agitation by Out-Pensioners for an improvement in their rates at the expense of the Royal Hospital caused Gladstone to convene another Committee under Lord Morley, 'to inquire whether the system of in-pensioners, as now in operation at Chelsea and Kilmainham, is more beneficial to the pensioner himself and a greater prospective boon to the deserving soldier than a system of out-pensions equal in cost to the country.' It was an absurd equation, as the 1870 Inquiry had conclusively shown; and since neither the previous arguments nor the earlier arithmetic had changed, the Committee arrived at the same conclusion and once again the Royal Hospital was reprieved. Among his formal recommendations – none of which were adopted – Lord Morley proposed the transfer of the administration of out-pensions from Chelsea to the War Office. It was something that should have been done two hundred years before. A further seventy years were to pass before the principle was finally accepted.

The third and last inquiry had a more curious origin. A retired Master-Gunner, Mr W. Punter of Portsmouth, founder and President of the resoundingly named 'Royal Chelsea Hospital Army Age Pensioners' Association' had addressed a lengthy statement to the Secretary of State for War, setting out a demand for an old age pension to be paid to retired soldiers in addition to their service or disability pensions and seeking to prove that the closing down of the Royal Hospital and the realization of its considerable assets would produce a fund sufficient to provide 14,575 of the oldest Out-Pensioners with an additional 6*d.* a day.

The worthy Mr Punter had done a great deal of homework, even to paying Messrs. Penney and Clark of Southsea to value the Hospital properties – at a figure of £2,323,500. He further argued – quoting the 1870 Report in evidence – that since the Hospital property had been bought out of deductions from army pay, it belonged in effect to the Out-Pensioners.

In some confusion, a Committee of Inquiry was hastily convened under Lord Belper and the now well-worn arguments were taken down, dusted, and deployed again, although this time enlivened by the evidence of Mr Punter, which, when it was not humorous, was frankly impertinent.

The Committee paraded a formidable array of witnesses, including the Senior Surveyor of the Office of Works, who countered Mr Punter's figures with a valuation of £977,377 for the Chelsea property. But the cream of the evidence is that provided by the In-Pensioners themselves and their forthright observations provide us with a delightful – and often pathetic – insight into the minds and characters of these old soldiers. Here are some extracts:

James Hayes, late 10th Hussars
'Are you comfortable at Chelsea? – I am comfortable enough, but there are a lot of disagreeable people there; I mean the private soldiers, the other pensioners. They watch you to see what you say and where you go, and then they report you to the non-commissioned officers and you get brought up before the Officers if you are caught napping.'

William Brown, late 72nd Regiment
'Are you comfortable in the Hospital? – I have nothing much to complain of, but of course having my wife outside, it makes my life what I may call a little bit miserable.'

John Thom, late 70th Foot
'Would you go out if you only got another 1/– a day? – Yes, I think I would. The inmates feel the draughts in the hospital, they give us such colds.'

John Burton, late St Helena Regiment
'I beg of you, in the name of all the pensioners, that you will deal liberally with us if you decide to break up the Hospital.'

John Whelan, late 101st Regiment
'Are you comfortable in the Hospital? – Yes, but it is a very strange place if once they get down on you. I was coughing and they were at me day and night and I did not know what to do with myself. You cannot tell who is your enemy, they baffle you so much.'

Charles Staker, late 4th Regiment
'Would you leave the Hospital if you could get another 2/– a day? – Yes, and be glad to do it.'

Hugh Wilson, late 79th Regiment
'Are you comfortable in the Hospital? – No, I cannot say I am. My place is up at the top and I have to go up 90 steps before I can sit down, and then if I want a smoke. I have to go down 180 steps to get one. From morning to night I go up and down at least 1080 steps. Getting upstairs tries me so.'

Joseph Farnham, late 20th Hussars
'It seems to me there is too much red tape. My rank, for instance, ought to be done away with because it causes a lot of jealousy my being a serjeant and such a young man (*32*).'

Frederick Fox, late 16th Lancers
'Have you many men under you who went out? – Yes, there was a man named Woods. He is the man you see now going about here begging with medals on.'

William Leaper, late 83rd Regiment
'Have you heard the suggestion that the Hospital may be done away with? – Yes, and I think it would be really terrible. I think the greater number would also say so and I hope I may never see it closed.'

Amery Coutts, late 64th Regiment
'Are you able to speak at all for any other men in your ward as to what their feeling is? – I do not know anything about them; it would take a wiser man than me to know the interior of those men.'

There, in the person of In-Pensioner Amery Coutts, speaks the authentic old soldier.

The Belper Committee might well have dragged on interminably, had it not been that on the fourth day, the Commander-in-Chief, H.R.H. the Duke of Cambridge, was called to give evidence. That peppery old gentleman strode briskly into action. Having demolished Mr Punter, he dismissed the Out-Pensioners' grievances as so much mutinous nonsense, hinted that the Queen might have something to say about the fate of her Royal Hospital (a shrewd body-blow, this), stated flatly that Chelsea existed to save old soldiers from dying in the workhouse, and declined to preside over its dismemberment.

After that, there was nothing left to say. In due course, the Committee published a muffled report, the main feature of which was a recommendation that the Royal Hospital might well be enlarged to accommodate a great many *more* deserving old soldiers.

Three times in twenty-five years, therefore, the fate of the Royal Hospital had hung in the balance. Three times a Committee had come to bury Caesar and ended up by praising him. The more one studies the lengthy evidence presented at each Inquiry the clearer it becomes that here was a victory of truth over prejudice. With very few exceptions the Governors and officers of the Hospital of that time were carefully non-committal. The case for the prosecution was always flimsy. Those who should have spoken vigorously for the defence preferred to swim with the tide; indeed, at least two eminent officers turned, as it were, Queen's Evidence. It was left to the In-Pensioners to fight their own battle for survival and this they did with a dignity and a sense of humour which together proved a formidable and, in the end, irresistible combination.

Meanwhile the village carried on much as it had always done. Rumour and gossip, as usual, must have supplemented the daily diet in the Wards, but the sound of thunder off-stage can have had small effect on the pattern of daily life.

The year 1885, shortly after the Morley report, provides us with a broad and illuminating picture of Chelsea at that period.

There were 531 In-Pensioners, 359 of them English, 117 Irish, 54 Scottish and 1 'Foreign'. Of these, surprisingly, only 261 had seen active service overseas – surprisingly, in view of the nation's long involvement in war. And of these again, 114 were Crimea veterans, 90 had fought in the Mutiny, and there remained one sole survivor of Waterloo. The slow decline of Waterloo veterans at the Royal Hospital is worth recording: in 1870 there were 53; in 1876 – 36; in 1878 – 11; in 1879 – 9; and finally in 1885 – 1. This grand old gentleman, Pte Heneage of the Inniskillings, died in 1890 at the age of 96.

The average age of In-Pensioners in 1885 was 62 years 9 months and all but seventeen were totally unfit for any kind of active employment.

The daily ration was contracted at 1*s*. 2*d*. per man and the cost of individual provisions – sober reading today – was as follows:

Beef	6*d*. per lb.
Mutton	5*d*. per lb.
Bacon	7½*d*. per lb.
Eggs	10*d*. per dozen
Butter	11*d*. per lb.
Cheese	6*d*. per lb.
Coffee	10*d*. per lb.
Cocoa	5*d*. per lb.
Milk	9¼*d*. per gallon
Ale and Porter	11*d*. per gallon

Remarkably, these prices – and the cost of the daily ration – *fell* dramatically during the depression of the 1890s.

Over in the Infirmary, business was brisk this year, for no fewer than 33,410 prescriptions were supplied compared with a figure of 17,027 ten years previously. And on April 17 the Physician and Surgeon triumphantly informed the Board that he had purchased Port Wine at 30s. instead of 36s. a dozen. He could have done better.

The Board were also driving hard bargains. In May they placed a contract with Sir Peter Tait & Co. for new great coats for all In-Pensioners at a cost of £672 1s., to be supplied in full by September. In fact they were delivered in batches, completing by March 31, 1886, whereupon the Board demanded compensation 'for the hardship incurred by those Pensioners who had waited in vain throughout the winter months'. Sir Peter Tait denied liability and pointed out that the contract was the least profitable into which he had ever entered. It availed him nothing and finally he made a cash reduction of £17 1s. which was distributed to thirty-eight chilly, deprived – but highly delighted old soldiers.

So the Victorian Age drew to its close, and with its passing was forged the first link with the village of to-day; for in 1902 the first South African veterans were admitted to the Royal Hospital. Seventy-two years later there are still seven In-Pensioner survivors of that distant war. When they enlisted, a motor-car was still a thing of wonder. They have lived to see men walk on the surface of the moon. Twice in their lifetimes they have seen the human race come close to self-extinction. Fortunately they will never know whether it is more successful at the third attempt. Their ages total 658 years – and that is a grand and honourable figure to record.

II

The forgotten Village

❦

A Second Interlude

On August 10, 1912, General Sir Neville Lyttelton was appointed Governor of the Royal Hospital. He presided over the In-Pensioners for nineteen years until his death in 1931, at the age of 85 – the last Governor to be appointed for life.

For thirty years the Hospital had been passing through one of its periodic phases of neglect. It had, in effect, become the forgotten village. A senior citizen who visited it, as a boy, during the summer of 1908, has recorded his impression:

> 'Over the whole place there was a curious atmosphere of desolation. Paintwork everywhere was chipped and peeling, the grass unkempt and the courtyards untended. This contagion of neglect had also infected the Pensioners, for they seemed lethargic and unmilitary, their uniforms shabby and soiled. They looked as if no one cared about them and – which was worse – as if they no longer cared about themselves.'

It is a strange commentary on our national character that the Royal Hospital should have entered upon so marked a decline during a period of unparalleled prosperity; and in this it was not alone.

Since the South African War, the Army as a whole had become a public Cinderella, starved of money and treated with the same disregard which had marked the years which followed the Crimean War. There are many In-Pensioners today whose enlistment dates from this period. They joined, as soldiers have always done, for many different reasons; boredom, poverty, the glamour of uniforms, the prospect of adventure and of travel to distant corners of Empire. Two even joined by mistake. But in their own working-class environment they were neither heroes nor even objects of pride. To 'go for a soldier' was widely held to be the last resort of wastrels and layabouts and the same public which had waved flags and cheered the 'Soldiers of the Queen' as they left to fight the Boers now turned its back on the soldiers of the King.

Even 'a shilling a day' proved to be a false prospectus, for by the time stoppages had been deducted, a man was lucky to have 2d. in his pocket. In-Pensioner Turp chuckles as he remembers: 'Miscellaneous stoppages! We used to say: "Just you wait until we get our hands on that Miss Cellaneous! We'll strangle her!"' And at Chelsea, in 1908, the 'peculiar money' of ordinary In-Pensioners was 7*d*. a week, a penny less than it had been in 1692 when the Hospital opened.

But the men in the ranks had two friends at court; Rudyard Kipling, who knew and understood them and who gave powerful and articulate expression to their sense of service and patriotism, and R. B. Haldane whose army reforms were even more radical and far-reaching than those of Edward Cardwell. This volunteer army – in that, at least, it had a moral superiority over French and German conscripts – would not have to wait long before it was given the opportunity to confound its critics.

Before General Lyttelton could set in train his own reforms at Chelsea, the nation was at war. The scale of that war and its unprecedented casualties created insuperable problems in the management of out-pensions and in 1916 the Ministry of Pensions was formed to administer all awards for disability. The Hospital establishment remained at its maximum figure of 558, but because of the sheer numbers involved, no war casualties were admitted between January, 1915 and March, 1919, and the minimum age for entry was fixed at 55, as it remains today.

On February 16, 1918, the war came to Chelsea. In one of the last German air-raids on London, a 500-lb. bomb destroyed the North-East wing of Light Horse Court, then in occupation by officers and staff of the Hospital. Capt. Ludlow, Captain of Invalids, his wife and three members of their family were killed, and four other members of the staff seriously injured. It was a moment of supreme irony; and it was not the last.

With the end of the war, the old order had gone for ever, obliterated in the futile slaughter of the Somme and in the mud of Passchendaele. An entire generation had all but vanished and of those who remained, every second man was now an old soldier. They had been promised a land fit for heroes. They were soon to discover that the reality was quite otherwise, and that the anonymous lady had been nearer the mark when she wrote to Charles II '. . . for, saie the people, when the wars is over, we are slited lik dogs'.

The 1920s were to be one of the strangest periods in the long and capricious story of the Royal Hospital.

During these years the first real programme of modernization since the buildings were taken into use was set in train. This was in some respects a matter of absolute necessity for the fabric of the Hospital had fallen into a melancholy state of disrepair and had immediate steps not been taken, it would have become virtually uninhabitable. The first work to be put in hand was the rebuilding of the bombed North-East wing, completed in 1922 to Wren's original design. When, by an astonishing coincidence, the same wing was destroyed again, it was to take not four, but *twenty* years for re-building to be completed. It would have taken even longer, but for the unorthodox intervention of the then Governor, General Sir Frank Simpson.

Early in 1920, a new bath-house was constructed in the East wing next to the choir vestry – cleanliness and godliness seem always to have rubbed shoulders at Chelsea – and later the same year, work began on the complete external redecoration of the buildings. But 1925, above all, was a year to remember for it saw the installation of electric lifts in the East and West wings. Of all the improvements and embellishments at the Royal Hospital, this surely was the most notable and the most gratifying. Wren, especially, with his constant care and consideration for the old soldiers' comfort, would have been delighted. So, too, would the sorely-tried, pipe-smoking In-Pensioner Wilson of pious memory.

Finally on August 8, 1929, the Board approved the installation of central heating throughout the whole Hospital. More had been achieved for the In-Pensioners' creature comforts in ten years than in the whole previous two and a half centuries.

Yet as so often in the past at Chelsea the left hand of authority seems neither to have known nor cared what the right hand was doing, and the In-Pensioners – despite the many structural improvements to their village – were largely left to their own devices. The spirit of the time is best summed up by the advice of a Lieutenant-Governor to a newly-arrived Captain of Invalids: 'Don't bother too much about the In-Pensioners and don't let them bother you.' It was hardly the best recipe for a happy and efficient village. And it may well have been this same Lieutenant-Governor of whom the following anecdote has survived. Walking along the Colonnade in civilian clothes, he passed four In-Pensioners seated on a bench, none of whom stood up or saluted. The conversation proceeded thus:

'Don't you know who I am?'
'No.'
'I'm the new Lieutenant-Governor.'
The four old soldiers studied him closely.
'Well,' said one eventually, 'you've got a nice job if you don't get drunk and lose it.'

It was, at this period, a village of very old soldiers – in 1924 there were still eleven survivors of the Crimean War and fourteen veterans of the Mutiny. Ashanti, Zululand, Afghanistan, Burma, Sudan, China – the medals of the In-Pensioners of the 1920s told their own story of distant battles now relegated by the traumatic years of 1914–18 to a lost limbo. In 1925 there were 182 South Africa men in the Hospital, and they, by comparison, were youngsters; yet even they seemed hardly to belong to the new, abrasive post-War world. They had indeed become forgotten men in a forgotten village, presided over by a kindly but ageing Governor who in his later years might be seen in public from time to time in an invalid chair. One single item from the archives of this period illustrates better than anything else the wind of change that was blowing through the land. On March 24, 1927 an abortive proposal was submitted to the Governor that 'direct representatives of the rank and file or of disabled ex-servicemen should be appointed to the Board of Commissioners.' It was the nearest anyone has got to a Royal Hospital Trade Union.

We last left the Irish In-Pensioners of the Royal Hospital at Kilmainham 250 years ago. They have been ill-served by later chroniclers, partly because, as servants of the British Crown, they were treated with little respect and less affection by most of their fellow-countrymen, and partly because their institution escaped the kind of public scandals which disfigured the conduct of affairs at Chelsea. We have seen that two attempts were made to close the establishment down in the nineteenth century and by 1853 the numbers had fallen to 140.

The 1921 Treaty which established the Irish Free State, and the subsequent disbanding of the old Irish regiments during the following years, marked the end of Kilmainham. The numbers were allowed to run down until on March 14, 1929, when the total of In-Pensioners had fallen to thirty-eight, the Army Council closed the Hospital. The remaining old soldiers were offered three alternatives:

1. Reversion to out-pension
2. Transfer to Chelsea
3. Free board and lodging in a civilian hospital or old people's home.

In the event, ten men elected to be transferred to Chelsea. So far as can be established from the records, the last of these was Thomas Brett, aged 82, of the Royal Irish Fusiliers – and he, being a good Irishman, departed not with a whimper but a bang, dismissed to out-pension on November 16, 1945 for 'serious misconduct' (unspecified).

Today the old Hospital building has become a repository for the *disjecta membra* of the National Museum of Ireland. It stands a stone's throw from Kilmainham Jail; and that seems not entirely inappropriate.

And then came the Great Depression. It reached into every corner of the land and infected every aspect of national life. In 1931 Macdonald's National Government was formed and against a background of massive unemployment the largely forgotten National Economy Act, cutting salaries by 10 per cent, was passed. It was the year of Noel Coward's *Cavalcade* and of Walton's *Belshazzar's Feast*. Stainforth flew an aeroplane at 407 m.p.h. and Whipsnade Zoo was opened. It was a year of crisis and contradiction.

The economy axe fell with only a gentle thud on the Royal Hospital, for during 1931 £32,000 was spent on maintenance of buildings alone. And with that curious streak of perverseness which has been a characteristic of Chelsea over the centuries, the Board chose this delicate moment to increase In-Pensioners' 'peculiar money'. Colour-Sergeants went up by a third from 7s. 6d. to 10s. a week while at the other end of the scale Privates' pay was trebled from 7d. to 1s. 9d. a week. It was long overdue, but with 3,000,000 men in the dole queues it is perhaps fortunate that the Board's action was not public knowledge.

178

Out of the economic crisis grew another and more dangerous
crisis of national morale, demonstrated by the growth of pacificism;
and during the 'Thirties a noticeable gulf developed between the
In-Pensioners at Chelsea and the public outside. This was partly a
reflection of the times, partly due to a lack of firmness on the part of
the Hospital staff, and partly the result of the public activities of a
small but significant number of In-Pensioners. George Downie, an
old soldier now in his eighties, describes his own reaction:

'In 1933 I had been out of work for virtually three whole years.
I had served throughout the Great War and had been wounded
at Messines and at Arras and since I had a small disability pension
I was not allowed to draw the dole. The only entertainment I
could afford was to take my wife out to a pub in Fulham for a
couple of hours on a Saturday night. Each Saturday a group of
three or four Chelsea Pensioners used to come into the pub
scrounging for free drinks. The men there would have nothing to
do with them, but they always found a blowsy old bag who was
good for a couple of pints. It really annoyed me and my wife to
watch them going through their act, knowing that they had the
best of everything back at Chelsea and not a care in the world.'

It was a reputation which, quite unfairly, was to pursue Chelsea
Pensioners whenever they walked abroad and it took many years to
live it down. The Chelsea Board at that period seems not to have
cared. Bill Townsend, who was appointed a Captain of Invalids in
1936 and who today after thirty-eight years is the longest-serving
member of the Hospital staff, recalls that Board meetings were
reputedly spent in swapping dubious stories and that on one
occasion a shorthand-typist was summoned from the Quartermaster's office to record some of the choicer examples for general
circulation. It was not the Royal Hospital's finest hour.

During the Munich crisis of 1938 the Board seems suddenly to
have woken up to the potential danger to the Hospital from enemy
air attack. Its anxiety took the odd form of an inquiry to the Ministry
of Works regarding the adequacy or otherwise of existing fire
insurance on the buildings. The Department duly put a price of
approximately £1,000,000 on 'rebuilding the Hospital with heating
and lighting installations'. It then proceeded to let a small cat out of

the bag, for its report continued: 'In the light of the recent Treasury paper on the subject, we should point out that if the Royal Hospital were destroyed, the probable likelihood is that no attempt would be made to rebuild it on its present scale, but a smaller and more convenient scheme at much less cost would be devised.' This interesting revelation seems to have surprised the Board as much as anyone; but the wheels of Whitehall grind slowly and before any further action – even in respect of fire insurance – developed, the country was at war.

The 1938 crisis had fortunately alerted the War Office and the Chelsea staff. Even with the available lifts, the evacuation of old and infirm men from the upper floors during air-raid alerts would have been virtually impossible (in 1939 there were still nine In-Pensioner survivors of the Zulu War of 1879) and accordingly plans had been made to move the whole establishment to Herefordshire. But the Governor, General Sir Harry Knox, would have none of it: 'My pensioners,' he announced, 'will not desert their posts in the face of the enemy. If necessary, I will form them up and march them down the King's Road to put heart into the people!' In the event some fifty of the oldest pensioners, together with a skeleton staff, were sent to Rudhall near Ross-on-Wye shortly before the outbreak of war; and the rest soldiered on at Chelsea.

Graham Dean was Adjutant at the Royal Hospital throughout the war years and he has left a moving record of how the old soldiers fared during the bombing of London. Shelters were improvised in the cellars under the Great Hall and the Chapel (a far cry from those carefree days of tippling and bawdy songs two hundred years before) and those men who could not be thus accommodated moved into the ground-floor wards. The old soldiers suffered greatly and during this period the mortality rate doubled.

The Hospital was an obvious target, sandwiched as it was between Chelsea Barracks and Battersea power station; and it got its fair share of attention. The first major structural damage was caused on October 26, 1940 when the third of a stick of four bombs destroyed the main staircase in the East wing (the scars are still to be seen).

On the night of April 16, 1941 a land mine destroyed the East wing of the Infirmary killing four nurses, the wardmaster and eight pensioners, including one centenarian, and injuring several others. The remainder of the Infirmary building was so badly damaged that the surviving patients had to be evacuated to civilian hospitals and later to Ascott House near Leighton Buzzard. Sir John Soane could never have imagined that his Infirmary would one day be in the firing-line and it is a tragic irony that so many old veterans who had survived the battlefields of Flanders, should have died at the hands of the same enemy in their quiet retreat at Chelsea.

After the destruction of the Infirmary, a further forty In-Pensioners were evacuated to Moraston House near Ross-on-Wye, and apart from sporadic incidents the next four years were largely uneventful – until January 3, 1945. At 8.50 a.m. that morning a V.2 rocket destroyed the North-East wing in Light Horse Court, killing Major Napier, the Physician and Surgeon, Capt. Bailey, a Captain of Invalids, two other residents, and an In-Pensioner who was standing in the Chapel. Nineteen other people were injured. It was the ultimate irony, for the rocket fell at almost the precise point where a German bomb had destroyed the same wing in February, 1918. The arm of coincidence could stretch no further.

Dean sums up the legacy of those embattled years thus:

> 'This proved to be the last incident of the war at the Royal Hospital, during which a land mine, a rocket, fourteen H.E. bombs and ten others that failed to explode, three anti-aircraft projectiles and over 100 incendiary bombs had fallen in the grounds, causing the deaths of twelve pensioners, seven members of the staff, and two other residents. Excluding cases of shock, thirty-three other persons were injured, so that casualties, exceeding 10 per cent of the numbers in residence, were comparable with those suffered by units on active service.'

So peace came; and the Royal Hospital had survived its greatest crisis. Now it had its own honourable scars to set beside those of its In-Pensioners. Wren would have been greatly saddened; but he would also have been very proud.

12
Phoenix from the ashes

Thus, as the war in Europe drew to its close, the Royal Hospital stood in disarray, the buildings scarred and disfigured and many of the In-Pensioners dispersed to the kindly but alien shelter of out-stations in the country. With the destruction of the North-East wing, admissions to the Hospital had been suspended so that by 1947 the numbers had fallen to 292, the lowest figure in its history.

In the scale of priorities of post-war reconstruction, the Hospital ranked a long way down the list. National resources, strained by the long years of war, were largely directed towards the provision of homes and other essential building, while at the same time the Labour Government embarked on the first stages of a vast and costly social revolution. For the In-Pensioners who remained at Chelsea, it was a time of improvisation which they accepted with the good humour and ribald comment of their kind. They had little alternative.

The most urgent problem arose from the destruction of the Infirmary, and the treatment of sick and infirm pensioners necessitated a variety of expedients such as admission to civil hospitals (themselves seriously overstrained) and transfer to those out-stations to which so many old men had been dispersed during the war.

As early as 1946 discussions had begun regarding the construction of a new Infirmary. The Ministry of Works favoured the derelict site of Sir John Soane's old building, chiefly because there was no immediate alternative other than Ranelagh Gardens, a suggestion that had already been mooted – and turned down – 140 years earlier. It must be remembered that at this date, service pensions were still being administered from Chelsea and the area to the east of Light Horse Court was occupied by temporary accommodation to house clerical staff. It was not until 1955 that the transfer of pensions to government departments released this ground for other purposes; and here, six years later, the new, superbly equipped Infirmary was opened on February 22 by Queen Elizabeth the Queen Mother. The decision to leave the old bomb-site in the North-West corner at least

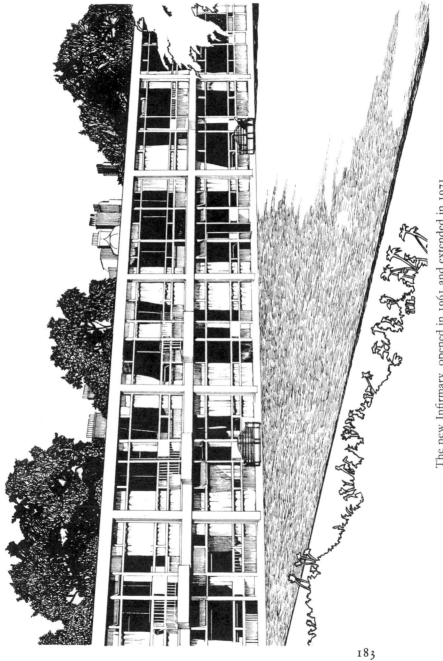

The new Infirmary, opened in 1961 and extended in 1971

temporarily derelict was both fortunate and wise, for in due course it was to produce a rich windfall for the Hospital funds.

In the spring of 1947, the pensioners who had been dispersed to Ascott House and Moraston House were transferred to the Royal School for the Blind at Leatherhead, which thus became effectively the Infirmary annexe of the Royal Hospital; and later in the same year, admissions were resumed. The post-war establishment still stood at its maximum of 558 (it was not reduced to its present total of 482 until 1972), but the residue of war damage and post-war austerity meant that the long waiting-list – the first for many years – could only be absorbed gradually. By 1951, however, the figure of In-Pensioners, including those at Leatherhead, had risen to 480; their average age was 72.

A Board Minute of January 25 of that year is of particular interest for it sets out in round figures the annual cost of running the Hospital and the individual cost of an In-Pensioner during the previous twelve months (1950).

The net cost was £172,000. Of this total £52,000 represented repairs and maintenance of buildings (the massive programme of modernization was yet to come), leaving a total of £120,000 to cover all in-pension charges.* This figure in turn was reduced further by the surrender of out-pensions so that the cost of an individual In-Pensioner worked out at £3 9s. 6d. a week (the Governor, be it noted, was *still* drawing £500 a year!). The same Minute also records that the cost of a bed in the Infirmary at Leatherhead was £255 a year, and the net cost of a patient £4 2s. a week.

On October 27, 1949, General Sir Bernard Paget was appointed Governor. It was to prove perhaps the most significant date in the whole history of the Royal Hospital.

General Paget had been C-in-C, Home Forces during the latter years of the war, and with the collapse of Italy and the final assault on *Festung Europa*, he had been appointed C-in-C, Middle East. Thus, at his retirement, this soldiers' soldier had been denied his life's ambition – to hold a major command in the field at the climax

---

* In 1784, at the date of Burke's Pay Office Act the equivalent figure was £29,512; in 1894, the date of the Belper Committee, it was £26,696; and in 1935, £35,112.

of the war. Military historians have paid him little honour. The high standing and present esteem in which the Royal Hospital is held are his lasting memorial; and he is remembered today at Chelsea with respect, affection – and awe. Looking back over the years, the Governor whom he most closely resembles is Sir George Howard, for in him were joined the same virtues of compassion and severity – virtues which the Hospital needed as never before when he came to preside over it.

One who knew him well has described him thus:

'Bernard Paget was a man out of context with his time. Ascetic (he had the appearance of a mediaeval abbot), deeply religious, he could be difficult (so could Churchill) and occasionally spiteful (so could De Gaulle). He would have made a splendid Parliamentary general under Cromwell; equally, light infantryman that he was, he would have stepped comfortably into Sir John Moore's shoes in the Peninsula. He was a kindly man and a strict disciplinarian – qualities which, in nice proportion, were and always will be the proper recipe for handling old men in general and old soldiers in particular. He was, quite simply, a great man; and like all great men, he himself took some handling.'

Lt. Gen. Sir William Oliver, who was Paget's Chief of Staff in the Middle East, has added his own gloss:

'He (Paget) had a built-in defence mechanism. He never called me by my Christian name the whole time I served with him – or anyone else by theirs (except his A.D.C.). Some years later I was dining with him at Ashridge Park, and after dinner he said: "Bill, will you have a glass of port?" I was completely taken aback. "General," I said, "that's the first time you've ever called me by my Christian name." He smiled. "I know," he said, a trifle sadly, "but in war it's easier to change a C.G.S. than a Bill."

'His great love was the British soldier and his whole life was dedicated to that great man. I have seen him light up like a torch and literally glow when some mention was made of an action or an event which showed the soldier at his best.'

General Paget's detractors – few but vocal – have argued that he was fortunate in the timing of his appointment which coincided with the relaxation of many post-war restrictions. As well suggest that Moses arrived on the shores of the Red Sea at a moment of providentially low tide! He was a stubborn and determined man who found the Royal Hospital at a low point in its fortunes and who, so to speak, took it by the scruff of the neck and shook it back to life. He was a bonny fighter against bureaucracy, and he once said – not altogether tongue in cheek – that he would readily burn down half the Hospital, if he could then use the insurance money to revitalize the other half. In the event, he achieved much of his purpose without resorting to arson.

By the spring of 1950, the problem of the two main areas of war damage at the Royal Hospital had become involved in that most intricate of labyrinths – the departmental committees of Whitehall. Wise old soldier that he was, General Paget therefore decided to conduct a holding operation against this deeply-entrenched redoubt, while switching his main attack to less easily defended positions. And his first objective was In-Pensioners' accommodation.

For nearly three hundred years, the Long Wards had remained unchanged except for the introduction of central heating and the installation of proper sanitary arrangements. Pensioners meals still came up from the Great Kitchen to be re-heated (sometimes) on the old ranges; and the old soldiers' berths, unaltered from 1692, still measured six-feet square. To this surviving anachronism the Governor now addressed himself, and progressively, from 1951 onwards, the berths in each of the Long Wards were enlarged to measure 6 feet by 9 feet. It may not sound particularly lavish, but the result was to increase the area of each berth by 50 per cent and to provide enough room for each pensioner to have a wardrobe, a chest-of-drawers and a writing table, and to dispense with the impersonal clutter of chests and presses in the ward corridors. Above all, it must have showed the old men that a new spirit of care and consideration was at work.

General Paget next turned his attention to the old and vexed question of In-Pensioners' recreation. Since Lord John Russell's time, the Great Hall had been closed for central messing and had been used as a reading room and a centre for communal meeting and relaxation. It had been the most contentious of Russell's reforms and entirely contrary to the 'collegiate' intention of Stephen Fox and Christopher Wren; and it had been the source of many problems – and abuses – as a result of ward feeding. Paget now proceeded to kill two birds with one stone. If he could provide some alternative accommodation for social activities, then he could free the Great

Hall for reversion to its original purpose as a communal refectory. And this he now did.

The origin of the In-Pensioners' Club is described in General Sir Frank Simpson's final Annual Report – thus:

'Before and during the 1939–45 war, an In-Pensioner's pay was only 1/9d a week and very few had the Old Age Pension which was 10/– a week. Consequently the problem of pocket money and the few luxuries it could buy was important in an In-Pensioner's mind. Some of the more fortunate ones made money by selling flowers and vegetables from their gardens. Those not so fortunate and who liked a glass of beer used to frequent the Chelsea pubs, and fumble in their pockets; and as these tricks became well-known in Chelsea, they used to venture further afield to the West End where the fumbling always worked! As, however, the Pensioners had very little spare cash, there was no object in having a Club, as opposed to a reading room, in the Royal Hospital, for the expenditure of the In-Pensioners would not have justified the overheads.

'In 1941, a detachment of In-Pensioners was sent to Moraston House, and as Moraston was situated several miles from the nearest pubs in Ross-on-Wye, a small canteen was started and proved to be very successful. Even during the war time beer shortage, the brewers made special deliveries to Moraston House.

'In 1947, the Infirmary was moved to Leatherhead from Ascott House and was joined there by the detachment from Moraston.

'At Leatherhead, Major Burrows, the Captain of Invalids in charge, having heard about the success of the Moraston canteen, started a club. As this prospered the then Governor, General Sir Clive Liddell, gave permission for a similar venture at Chelsea. In 1948 a small Club was started in one of the In-Pensioners' Ward extensions in No. 6. Light Horse Court [*beer only and port for NCOs!*]. This, too, was so successful that in 1952 General Sir Bernard Paget authorized the opening of the present Club in what had been the NCOs' Billiard Room.'

From little acorns, great oaks grow; and under the lively guidance, first of the Adjutant, Brigadier Cuddon, and then of R.S.M. Ives, the In-Pensioners' Club prospered greatly, with the addition of an elegant Ladies' Room and an astonishing turnover, in 1972, of £58,000.* Given the convivial propensities of old soldiers, its

* This was appreciably more than Wren's entire expenditure on building Figure Court, including the Great Hall and the Chapel.

financial success was never in doubt; but that is perhaps the least of its contributions to the new image of the Royal Hospital. For the first time in three centuries, it provided a proper social centre for the village. Here the In-Pensioners could entertain – and be entertained – in a setting which would have greatly pleased Matthew Ingram. To use a modern euphemism, it solved at a stroke one of the age-old problems of this age-old village.

It also solved half of General Paget's problem of creating a truc sense of community among his old soldiers. He now acted upon the natural corollary.

The Club had put the old recreation room in the Great Hall out of business. More importantly, it had made possible the revival of an old tradition – and Bernard Paget was a convinced traditionalist. He, of all men, had read and understood Charles's Royal Warrant. So, in 1955, after extensive reconstruction of the Great Kitchen, the Great Hall was reopened for central messing. As one In-Pensioner has touchingly put it: 'It was as if one of the old glories had returned.'

It was a shrewd psychological decision for it re-created the old quasi-regimental sense of community, removed the occasion for one of the oldest Hospital abuses, and, quite incidentally, improved dramatically the whole standard of messing. It also made good economic sense.

We may recall that many years previously the kindly Governor, Sir George Howard, had issued an instruction 'that action be taken . . . to take food to those in the Wards who are too infirm to help themselves and who have grown grey in the Service of their King and Country'. So it is today; for meals are served in Nos. 1 and 2 Wards to those In-Pensioners who, 'grown grey in the Service of their Queen and Country' are too infirm to make their way to the Great Hall. Sir George Howard would have approved.

In these ways, General Paget set in train the grand revival of the Royal Hospital. Each of his three major reforms – the enlarging of the berths, the establishment of the Club, the renaissance of the Great Hall – had a single purpose: to recreate in this royal and ancient institution a sense of corporate pride and corporate contentment. The In-Pensioners themselves were to prove harder nuts to crack.

Discipline and pride in appearance were both in short supply when General Paget came to Chelsea. The decline in standards was by no means general but there were enough black sheep in the flock to give renewed colour to the old pre-war reputation of the pensioners. Paget was a martinet, unexcelled as a trainer of soldiers, yet – perhaps through innate shyness – awkward in his attempts to communicate with the men under him. He was quick to realize that the In-Pensioners required a different approach to a battalion of light infantrymen, but less quick to appreciate that the Royal Hospital was not Cowley Barracks. So it was that a curious paradox arose. While the Governor pressed ahead with his imaginative reforms, many of the old abuses – the disposal of rations and the selling of clothing – flourished without check; the old demon that had bedevilled the Hospital since its earliest days still stalked the Colonnade and the guardroom did some exceedingly brisk business – until the appointment in 1954 of Jimmie Ives.

R.S.M. Ives was a retired warrant-officer of the East Surreys. Captured by the Japanese at Singapore, he had spent four dark years in prison camps, including those on the infamous Siam railway, where he had learned all he needed to know about human nature. He was to serve the Royal Hospital under four Governors and become a familiar public figure as he led his twelve In-Pensioners into the Albert Hall each year at the Festival of Remembrance; and the smartness and bearing of those old gentlemen is the best of all tributes to the silent revolution which their R.S.M. worked at Chelsea. In 1954, the picture was very different.

Jimmie Ives well remembers his first Church parade and his astonishment at the appearance of the In-Pensioners. 'Those few who had troubled to clean their buttons had Brasso all over their scarlet. Really scruffy they looked.' And so he set to work.

He is the first to disclaim any exclusive credit, and this is true; for Bernard Paget's dedication to the Hospital and his own qualities of leadership and understanding were soon reflected in the staff around him. He had devoted himself to a revival of this great and honourable institution and that sense of devotion was contagious. There was no sickness at the heart of the Hospital that could not be cured by firmness and good humour and those were the specifics which Ives prescribed in his daily dealings with the pensioners; and they thrived on the treatment.

The place was full of 'characters'. Lt. Col. 'Stickie' Hill, who came to Chelsea as Quartermaster about the same time as Ives, recalls one memorable example.

In-Pensioner Monty Beart was a ladies' man – on a grand and uninhibited scale. Over a period of time he acquired a following of five elderly widows, who he played off against each other with Machiavellian skill. To each he presented himself as a man of property and to each he promised a share of his estate in gratitude for her kindness and consideration for an old and lonely soldier. In due course, In-Pensioner Beart took sick and died. The following morning five desolate ladies presented themselves at Col. Hill's office and demanded to see the old man's will. There was no will. And when In-Pensioner Beart's estate was wound up, his worldly possessions consisted of his uniforms (the property of the Royal Hospital) – and £1 os. 9d. in cash.

Not all were so scantily endowed. There was the old gentleman who, when he tired of Hospital routine and the mundane diet of the Great Hall, donned an elegant civilian suit and booked himself into the Ritz for a week, there to recharge his batteries in a more sophisticated setting.

Gradually, as the Club got into its stride and the Great Hall resumed its traditional role, a new spirit began to animate the Long Wards. It is well illustrated by the fact that, at the date of Sir Bernard Paget's retirement in 1956, the guardroom, for lack of customers, had gone out of business.

General Paget had found King Charles's 'noble charity' sunk in apathy and, in a sense, bleeding to death from wounds, of which some at least were self-inflicted. With patience and an almost puritan dedication he nursed it through its crisis so that when the time came for him to go, the Hospital was not only revived in body but transformed in spirit. As one of his successors has put it, 'he inherited an institution and made of it a home'. The In-Pensioners owe him an immeasurable debt.

In the following five years, under General Sir Cameron Nicholson, the great revival went forward. It is a measure of the new spirit abroad in the village that the daily routine of running the Long Wards – delegated to the pensioners themselves – had become so time-consuming (and so vital to the continuing sense of purpose and concern) that in 1958 a new grade was introduced and Sergeant-Majors were appointed for the first time in each Company. There was no shortage of qualified men, for among the In-Pensioners were many old soldiers who had served with distinction in the highest non-commissioned ranks.

Nonetheless, the job required then – as it does today – special qualities of tact and understanding. Hospital Sergeant-Majors cannot rely on the normal sanctions of military discipline, for the Royal Hospital is not a military institution,* and the pensioners are not subject to military law. In each Company there were, there are, and there always will be – as in any community – the withdrawn and the lonely, the cheerful and the extrovert, the amenable and the aggressive, the modest and the opinionated; in short, a fair cross-section of the human condition. To manage so diverse a group of old men requires the patience of Job, the wisdom of Solomon, and the professional expertise of a psychiatrist. It is probably true to say that latterly the quality of life at Chelsea has risen and fallen in direct proportion to the quality of its Company Sergeant-Majors.†

About this time, a small but memorable reform was introduced. After lengthy argument – the correspondence is a marvellous commentary on the British genius for making new molehills out of other molehills – War Office sanction was obtained for the wearing of anodized buttons on scarlet coats and blue waistcoats. It meant a soldier's farewell to button-sticks and Brasso. It also meant that R. S. M. Ives could face his Sunday Church parades without wincing.

Meanwhile, down in the forest of Whitehall something stirred. The question of building a new Infirmary had been discussed as long ago as 1946. It will be remembered that sick and infirm In-Pensioners had been accommodated at Leatherhead since 1947 and while this arrangement had served its temporary purpose, the position had become increasingly difficult as admissions to Chelsea began to swell the establishment. So long as service pensions were administered from Chelsea and the only suitable site for an Infirmary

* In fact the Royal Hospital is still technically a Garrison since its original classification has never been countermanded by Royal Warrant.

† On first appointment they were paid 17s. 6d. a week. The figure is now £1.75 a week.

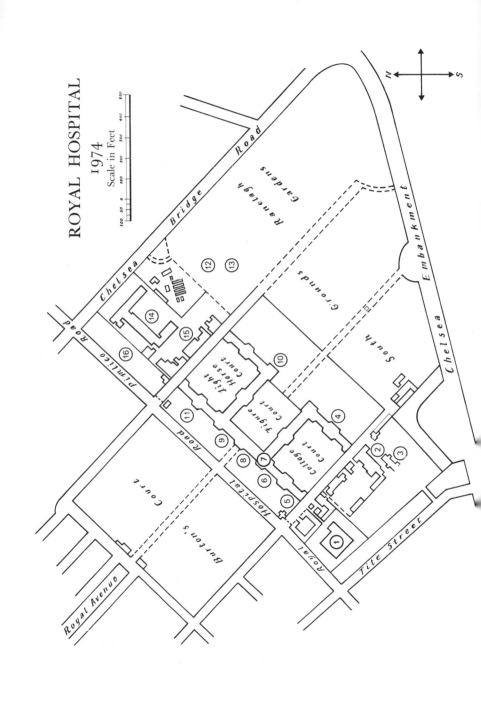

ROYAL HOSPITAL
1974
Scale in Feet

Key to Ground Plan of the Royal Hospital, 1974

1. National Army Museum, site of Walpole House and of Sir John Soane's Infirmary
2. Library and Roman Catholic Chapel, site of Sir John Vanbrugh's greenhouse and Orangery
3. Gordon House
4. Site of Chelsea College and Wren's Infirmary
5. In-Pensioners' Club
6. Former Officers' Hall
7. Great-Kitchen
8. Great Hall
9. Chapel
10. Governor's Residence and State Apartments
11. North-East Wing, twice destroyed by enemy action
12. Site of Ranelagh House
13. Site of the Rotunda
14. New Infirmary
15. Secretary's Office and Museum
16. Old Burial Ground

was still occupied by Nissen huts, the departmental committees had a copper-bottomed alibi for inaction. In 1955, however, the responsibility for service pensions was at last – *at long, long last* – transferred to Stanmore, and a splendid silence descended upon the hutment area. For three more years, the Treasury fought a stubborn rearguard action,* but finally in 1958 permission was granted for the site to be cleared. Early in 1959 a contract was placed and on June 25 the foundation stone was laid. At last the phoenix was rising from the ashes.

The decision to proceed with the building of the Infirmary seems to have acted like a catalyst on the spending departments. In 1958, thirteen years *post factum*, the Treasury also approved the re-building of the derelict North-East wing, although, as we shall see, words were to prove no substitute for action. A year later, a new ceiling was provided for the Great Hall and the Battle Honour panels were re-inscribed. In 1960, the Museum was opened in the Secretary's office block and new, enlarged lifts were installed in the East and West wings. The Hospital was alive with activity. It was a splendid moment to be an In-Pensioner.

In June, 1961, General Nicholson was succeeded by a man who was destined to leave upon the Royal Hospital a mark as indelible as that imprinted by Bernard Paget.

General Sir Frank Simpson shared with General Paget two characteristics: an absolute devotion to the Royal Hospital and a stubborn determination to puncture bureaucracy. There the similarity ended; for General Simpson was a most unusual soldier. In the first place, he had a very shrewd nose for administrative finance, a talent which was to pay at least one notable dividend; and he had an equally shrewd nose for public relations. Throughout his eight years at Chelsea, he set out to sell the Royal Hospital to the public, on the elementary principle that public opinion can be a formidable weapon against an entrenched Establishment. His technique took two forms.

First he took his old soldiers to the people. The Annual Reports

---

* Should any reader doubt the versatility of Treasury tactics, he may be interested to know that a suggestion was advanced that it might be cheaper to pull down the Royal Hospital than to build a new Infirmary.

during his Governorship list an extraordinary traffic of In-Pensioners: to public functions, to private parties, to royal occasions, to parish fêtes, to regimental reunions at home, to army stations abroad, singly or in coach-loads, by the odd couple to drink Guinness at Park Royal, by the dozen to give colour and meaning to Remembrance Day services up and down the country. R. S. M. Ives's Orderly Room became a regular tourist office.

Secondly, he brought the people to his old soldiers – particularly people who could and would be of service to the Royal Hospital; for, unlike Bernard Paget, he was a natural communicator, entirely at ease with his old gentlemen and in every sense the squire of his village.

But always he was himself an old soldier and like Sir George Howard he could both bark and bite. There are still many at Chelsea who ruefully recall the price of a moment's indiscretion. Bernard Paget may have been the counterpart of George Howard. General Simpson had no precursor. He was a great Governor and an 'original'.

Sir Frank Simpson's eight years at Chelsea were marked by four major events which were to set the seal upon the grand revival initiated by Paget.

With the opening of the new Infirmary, the future of the derelict site in what was to become known as 'the North-West corner' again came under discussion. For some time the National Army Museum, inadequately housed at Camberley, had been looking for a suitable London home. Accordingly, negotiations began for the acquisition of the old Infirmary site and the construction of a purpose-designed building. These negotiations were to drag on for six years during which Sir Frank Simpson displayed a bargaining skill and a tactical virtuosity which would have done credit to the toughest Trade Union official. One of the negotiators remembers: 'Simbo never missed a trick. He was always careful to read the small print – which was not surprising, since he wrote most of it himself.'

General Simpson found a worthy adversary in his old friend Field Marshal Sir Gerald Templer who was Chairman of the Museum Council and subsequently himself became a Chelsea Commissioner. Lord Ranelagh would have rather liked that. Eventually, on November 30, 1967, a 999 year lease was signed and Field Marshal

Templer handed to General Simpson a cheque for £160,000, representing the premium on the lease. This sum virtually doubled the existing Hospital funds. One can almost sympathize with Sir Robert Walpole, whose house had once occupied this site. He could have done with the money.

The Governor simultaneously turned his attention to the ruined North-East wing. As we have seen, Treasury approval for re-building had been given as far back as 1958, but no action had been taken until the autumn of 1961, when work was suspended within a few weeks of starting. On Founder's Day the following June, at which the Queen was Inspecting Officer, Sir Frank Simpson had this to say in his reply to the Royal address:

> 'Today over seventeen years after its destruction (the North-East wing) is still a ruin. Alas, although as planned the first work of reconstruction started last September, it was immediately called off owing to the cuts in capital expenditure which the government had to impose last year. You will appreciate what a disappointment to us this was. Our current waiting list is over 80. . . . There is therefore a real need for an increase in our accommodation.'

The Governor had judged his distinguished audience very nicely. Within an hour the Speaker of the House of Commons was asking the then Member for Chelsea whether he would like to raise the matter on an adjournment debate in the House. That debate was held within three weeks and was followed the next morning by a cogent leader in *The Times* urging that the withdrawn funds should be restored. They were; for, tucked away in the 1963 Annual Report is this item: 'Work was begun on the re-construction of the bomb damaged North-East wing.' It was completed two years later and was opened on January 24, 1966, to provide modern accommodation, half of it air-purified, for an additional sixty-four In-Pensioners.

1963 saw the rising of another phoenix, when the derelict shell of Vanburgh's eighteenth-century Orangery was restored to house a magnificent library and a Roman Catholic chapel. Of all the new features of these years of revival and renaissance at Chelsea they are perhaps the most imaginative and the most elegant.

There remained the fourth and last monument to Sir Frank Simpson's singleness of purpose. The new Infirmary, opened in 1961, contained eighty beds. Like Sir John Soane's original building, it had never been adequate to meet the demands of a village where the problems of geriatrics and the natural infirmities of old age would always put a growing premium on accommodation. For four years Sir Frank beat upon the gates of the Establishment and deployed his formidable artillery of persuasion against all and sundry until, on Founder's Day, 1968, he was able to announce that Treasury approval had been given to a forty-bed extension to the existing building. It was the last, and in some ways the greatest, of his many services to the Royal Hospital.

In June 1969, Sir Frank Simpson's tour of duty at the Royal Hospital ended. In the twenty years since Sir Bernard Paget took office the Royal Hospital had been transformed, the battered fabric restored, and the In-Pensioners had regained their pride and their self-respect. Many hands had contributed to this work of recovery, but none more so than the pensioners themselves. The sun had never shone more brightly on the village in Chelsea.

13
The Village to-day

The day is Easter Monday. The scene – the Cowdray Hunt Point-to-Point meeting. A hairy young person of indeterminate gender studies a group of scarlet-coated In-Pensioners with interest and obvious incomprehension. Presently the person approaches them. 'My friends and I were wondering. Are you Salvation Army?' A pause. Then up speaks In-Pensioner Green. 'Well, my dear, we certainly used to be Army, but we're long past all hope of salvation.'

It is not as uncommon a scene as might be supposed, for there are a surprising number of people – and not only of the younger generation – who do not recognize a Chelsea Pensioner when they see one; and that, despite the ubiquitous eye of the television camera. 'Look, dear,' said an elderly lady to her companion in a Truro café, 'those old men look just like Chelsea Pensioners.' 'Madam,' replied one old gentleman gallantly, 'we *are* Chelsea Pensioners.'

The bridge that Sir Frank Simpson built between pensioners and public has been greatly strengthened and secured. Forty or fifty years ago it was quite otherwise, for 7*d*., or even 1*s*. 9*d*., a week was hardly a passport to far-off places and for the most part In-Pensioners moved in the narrow circle of their village and its surroundings. Londoners knew them by sight. They also knew them by reputation – and kept their distance.

Today, as they respect themselves, so are the In-Pensioners respected, and their scarlet coats are greeted with pride, not untouched by nostalgia, up and down the country and as far afield as Paris and Berlin, Washington and Toronto. It is a strange paradox, for in a world of little Englanders, the In-Pensioners seem to epitomize the old grandeur and greatness. They first took the stage in a period of national revival and they have now become an honoured symbol of the old order at a time of national decline. Only in England could such a thing happen.

We have seen how their fortunes have changed across three centuries and how they have survived in spite of others – and sometimes in spite of themselves. Let us see how they are faring to-day.

Since 1847 the cost of maintaining the Royal Hospital has been borne out of public funds – the In-Pensioners themselves by the Ministry of Defence and the buildings and services by the Department of the Environment. In addition, the Commissioners dispose of substantial sums known under the general heading of the Army Prize and Legacy Fund, to which is added the income from rented Hospital property.* The Drouly Legacy, for example, largely pays for the upkeep of Ranelagh Gardens and the South Grounds, while also providing various amenities for the pensioners which are not covered by the Defence Vote; and at Christmas each pensioner receives 25p from the Ingram Legacy. It is a prosperous village and its inhabitants have good reason to remember with gratitude their 'pious founder' at each annual celebration of Founder's Day,† for they are better endowed today than he could ever claim to be.

The basic qualification for admission to the Royal Hospital is that a man should be in receipt of an army pension, whether for service or disability, that he should be of good character, reasonably fit, and have no relatives financially dependent upon him. The normal minimum age for entry is 65, but where a man can be shown to be incapable of earning his own living by reason of disability or infirmity, the minimum age may be reduced to 55.‡ In ordinary circumstances, no man is accepted if he is likely to be a permanent in-patient in the Infirmary, but in practice, the Governor is given wide discretion and each application is treated strictly on its merits. The criterion is a man's inability to earn his own living while still being generally capable of looking after himself.

A number of misapprehensions have arisen over the years. First,

---

* In 1973, this income amounted to £12,775. Under the existing licence, the Royal Horticultural Society pays an annual sum of £2,005 for the use of the South Grounds for the Chelsea Flower Show – and a surcharge for repairing subsequent damage!

† Founder's Day, celebrated without interruption since 1692, commemorates both the birthday of King Charles II and the occasion of his restoration, which fell upon the same date. On this, the high point of the Hospital year, the statue in Figure Court is garlanded and all In-Pensioners wear sprigs of oakleaf.

‡ In cases of disability resulting from army service, an applicant *can* be accepted at any age, but such exceptions are now very rare. Clearly there are disadvantages where a man may find himself surrounded by pensioners old enough to be his *grandfather*.

an applicant need not have served in the Regular Army. Provided he has a disability pension arising out of army service, he can have been a Territorial soldier or have served only during a period of hostilities. There are several such In-Pensioners. In theory, a man could enlist on Monday and be invalided out of the army through injuries received on Tuesday, and that could be sufficient qualification in due course for entry into the Hospital. Secondly, a man does not have to be a widower or a bachelor. If his disability – or infirmity – is such that his wife is unable to look after him, or if he is himself physically unable to care for an ailing wife, then subject to her agreement he may apply for admission. There are also several such In-Pensioners. If, however, after entry to Chelsea he wishes to marry, then he is obliged to revert to out-pension. And that, too, is not unknown. Not all old soldiers simply fade away.

At the end of our story we shall look at some of the reasons why so many Out-Pensioners are not attracted to the Royal Hospital. It is worth examining the other side of the coin.

Money is the least of motives. On retirement from civilian occupation, all eligible old soldiers today are in receipt of an old age pension and at least one form of army pension. Many have an additional civil pension or private means. On admission to Chelsea, they surrender their army pension, but retain all other sources of income, and the Hospital offers a wide variety of light occupations which provide additional pin-money. It is no longer by any stretch of imagination a paupers' home.

Some apply for admission because soldiering is in their blood and for them the Hospital is their natural retreat – 'my wife made me promise that, if she went first, I would come into Chelsea'. Others have tried – and failed – to make a home with their children. This works both ways. 'Dad's pension' can swell the household kitty – and old soldiers make good washers-up and baby-sitters. But they can grow old ungracefully, cantankerous, confused, and incontinent. Yet the young are often selfish and impatient and there have been instances of old and infirm men simply being dumped on a bench at Chelsea and left there by exasperated sons or daughters.

But the more one talks to In-Pensioners, the clearer it becomes that the greatest single reason why they come to Chelsea is the one infirmity of old age for which no easy cure has yet been found –

loneliness. Many such men enter the Hospital with strong feelings
of rejection, but only the most intractable – or wilful – fail to respond
to the atmosphere of kindness and good humour which surrounds
them on arrival. An applicant for the post of R.S.M. once asked
Jimmie Ives what the Chelsea job was all about. 'It's not difficult,'
he replied. 'Just be kind to the old men.' It is Matthew Ingram's old
and proved prescription.

New recruits* to the Royal Hospital are encouraged to spend a
few days at Chelsea taking the temperature of the water, so that they
can be sure that it is neither too hot nor too cold for their individual
taste. Once they make their decision to come in – and very few do
not – the Hospital assumes complete responsibility for them – food,
lodging, clothing, entertainment, and medical care. They pay not a
penny. As we have seen earlier, it costs the Hospital £152 to kit
each man out, and on average 42p a day to feed him. The quality and
variety of the diet would do credit to a high-class hotel. And the
medical facilities in the Infirmary are alone sufficient justification for
all old soldiers to think twice before dismissing the Royal Hospital
as an over-publicized poorhouse.

The underlying philosophy of life at Chelsea is that of voluntary
co-operation – a philosophy which might well serve as a touchstone
for industrial relations outside. Mavericks are rare, and use of the
ultimate sanction of expulsion against them rarer still. Discipline is
unobtrusive and no more than is necessary to maintain those
standards of behaviour and appearance which old soldiers would
themselves expect and demand, while compulsion extends only to
dress regulations; and to weekly church and pay parades. In-Pensioners have long applied their traditional ingenuity to get exemption from the former, while voluntary absenteeism from the latter
would be *entirely* out of character. For the rest, the old men are free
to come and go, whether in uniform or civilian clothes, and they
draw 25p a day ration allowance when absent on leave. One pensioner, after a lengthy sojourn with his daughter in Australia,
cheerfully collected £51.75p. Nor are creature comforts overlooked.
Each pensioner is entitled to draw one pint of beer a day from that

---

* The age of applicants has tended to rise in recent years. Early in 1974, the
average age of all In-Pensioners was 78, and the average age at death, a fraction
over 81. A hundred years ago, the equivalent figures were 62 and 73.

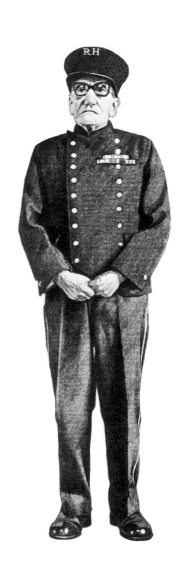

Double-breasted Button Waistcoat
I/P B. Turp, RVM, 1st Royal Dragoons

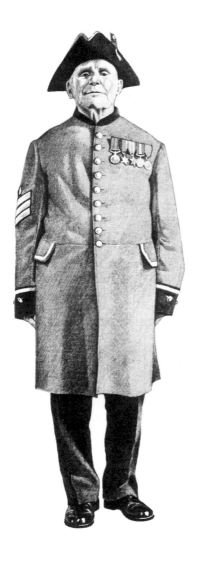

Ceremonial Scarlet
C/Sgt J. Blair, Scots Guards

202

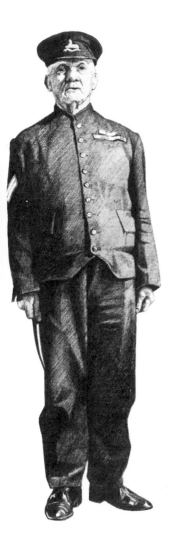

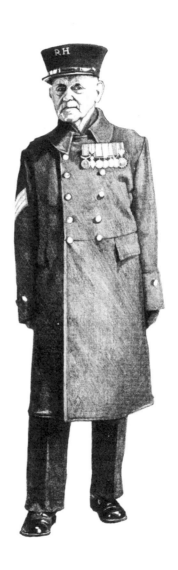

Blue Winter Greatcoat
Sgt G. Fordham, MM, RAEC

Single-breasted Lounge Waistcoat
Cpl W. Wildgoose, R. Lincolns

203

celebrated cellar below the Great Hall, and also a ration of forty cigarettes or 2 ounces of tobacco a week, a practice that goes back to the distant days of Matthew Ingram.

The old soldiers can demonstrate a remarkable range of craftsmanship and expertise, for they come, for the most part, from a world where automation was unknown and where a man's livelihood came from the skill of his own hands. Many, of course, come from those civilian employments such as the Corps of Commissionaires, War Department Police or the Post Office which have traditionally drawn on ex-servicemen; but a random sample from their record cards in 1972 threw up such widely differing talents as these:* jockey, valet, chauffeur, miner, publican, golf professional, tinsmith, dog-breeder, huntsman, hotelier, architect's draughtsman, saddler, gravedigger, housepainter, rat-catcher, market gardener, saxophonist, tax inspector, beadle, and bus-driver.

As a corollary to this 'ministry of all the talents', the Hospital is largely run by the In-Pensioners themselves. This has two advantages. Not only does it save a great deal of public money but it provides light and interesting paid employment for men who are sound in wind and limb and want to keep themselves occupied. Thus they act as 'home helps' to the officers of the Hospital (the word 'batman' is unpopular), librarians, museum attendants, chapel clerks, stewards in the Club, ushers of the Great Hall, and messengers. Some work in the grounds and greenhouses, or in the handicrafts section, while others cultivate their own allotments. No man need be idle. No man can be compelled to work.

What manner of men are the old soldiers of the Royal Hospital today, drawn as they are from every corner of these islands and from so many walks of life? To choose examples from so rich and diverse a field is invidious; but we will take two who are both typical – and typically different.

---

* In 1972 there were no fewer than sixty-eight former army bandsmen at the Hospital. They would have made a memorable sight – and sound – on parade.

We have already briefly met In-Pensioner Bertram Turp, born eighty-nine years ago at the Plough Inn in the Essex village of South Ockendon. The son of a dairyman and with no military tradition in his family, he determined from boyhood up 'to go for a soldier' and enlisted on St Patrick's Day, 1902 – 'they must have heard about me in South Africa, because two months later the war out there ended.' The circumstances of his enlistment illustrate the delightful vagueness of the would-be recruit. 'I wanted to soldier with horses. For me it was the cavalry or nothing. So they gave me a list of cavalry regiments and there at the top I saw "1st Dragoon Guards" and I thought: "That's good enough for me", and so I said I'd like to join the "1st *Dragoons*". Next thing I knew I'd been sent to the Royals at Shorncliffe. I'd never heard of them! But I'm not sorry the day I went to them. A lovely regiment.'

Bert Turp spent his first Christmas in the army on stable guard. 'I had my dinner on one bale of hay and I sat on another. When I got to the Christmas pudding, the horse in the next stall kept turning round and sniffing, so I said "Come on, mate, you try some", and he finished the lot, custard and all!'

But Christmas was something special, and Bert Turp remembers the wretched quality of normal army food and army cooking (although both were probably better than most men then enjoyed outside). 'We got a pound of bread a day and if you didn't put some of it away in your box, you had nothing left for tea.' Pay was notionally 1s. a day before stoppages. 'We had two pay days a week – 2s. on Tuesday and 3s. on Friday – and even that was usually docked again for barrack damages.' But he loved the life – the horses, the opportunities for sport, and the special ties that bound officers and men together in a cavalry regiment of the old army. To this day he retains a delightful snobbery – reminiscent of the old Light Horsemen of Chelsea two centuries ago – and his conversation is sprinkled with references to Debrett. 'I remember when Viscount Ednam....'

In 1904, the Royals sailed for India and Bert Turp was not to see England again for fifteen years, except briefly in 1914 *en route* for Flanders. He had long been fascinated by the blacksmith's trade – 'they always knew where to find me when I was a boy, up at the forge, feeding the jackdaws and watching the men at work' – and so in due course, he applied to become a shoeing-smith. 'You started as a cold shoer, a learner, but you got an extra 6d. a day, and I remember that when I qualified I got 1 year 11 days back pay! And that was a lot of money.' So the dairyman's son form South Ockendon became a farrier.

In 1911, the Royals moved to South Africa, first to Roberts' Heights in Pretoria and then to Potchefstroom. Bert Turp loved the country – 'wonderful climate, beautiful colours' – but was less enchanted with the Boers. In 1913, he was involved in the Johannesburg riots, a forgotten episode in which the Royals had to deal not only with civil violence but also with the redoubtable agitator Mrs Fitzgerald – 'a proper hell-cat, she was.' It was a new experience, soon to be overshadowed by events far away in Europe.

The outbreak of war brought the Royals back to Tidworth, where they re-equipped, collected their reservists, and, early in October, took ship for Zeebrugge. 'Our first night we bivouacked on Ostend racecourse. The next morning it was "Saddle up" at 3.30 and off to Ypres. We arrived there on October 13. We were to get to know the place pretty well during the next four years.

'When we got there, the town was still untouched, although we knew the Germans weren't far away. In fact, by an odd coincidence, our first brush was with the 24th German Dragoons – and we saw them off in double quick time.'

Bert Turp's war took its course for the most part uneventfully, although one suspects that he is typically reticent. 'I was at 1st, 2nd and 3rd Ypres and came through without a scratch, not even a cold in the head. And I kept my same black mare right through it all.' But fate had one trick up its sleeve for Shoeing-Smith – now Farrier-Sergeant – Turp.

On the morning of March 24, 1918 – with that astonishing recall of most old soldiers he remembers the time as 12.50 p.m. – he was with a mixed squadron of Royals, 10th Hussars and 3rd Dragoon Guards at Collezy. Let him tell the story himself:

'We were gathered in a sunken road when the order came to draw swords and to hold them down along our horses' shoulders so the enemy wouldn't catch the glint of steel. Then we scrambled up the bank and the order came, "Right shoulder!" and we formed line to charge.

'We could now see the enemy for the first time – infantry in the open. We had always been taught that a cavalry charge was made six inches from knee to knee, but it didn't work out like that and we went off as if we were going round Tattenham Corner, yelling like mad.

'I rode straight for a German who was kneeling down. He fired at me and missed and my sword went through his neck and out the other side. Then I took another man on my near side through the shoulder and as my sword came clear I saw another German in front of me. He turned to run and I caught him in the backside which must have made him hop!

'It was all over very quickly and the retreating Germans ran into the 3rd Dragoon Guards who had got round into a wood behind them. The German casualties were about seventy killed and 100 prisoners (one of them told me had been a waiter at the Ritz in London). We had six killed and three officers and six men wounded and we lost several horses.'

It was probably the last cavalry charge of the war and for his conduct in it Farrier-Sergeant Turp was awarded the Meritorious Service Medal.*

So the war ended, and in 1923, on St Patrick's Day, the date on which he had enlisted, Staff-Sergeant Turp hung up his boots and his saddle for the last time, and departed into civilian life on a pension of £1 8s. a week.

After a while, he went as second horseman to the Colonel of his regiment, Major-General Burn-Murdoch, in the Quorn country of Leicestershire. But ex-Farrier-Sergeant Turp, who had gone through the war 'without even a cold in the head', found, as Hilaire Belloc had done, that the Midlands were 'sodden and unkind'; and on doctor's advice he returned to London where, with his Colonel's help, he got a job as a Keeper in the Royal Parks. He was to spend thirty-four years there in the Royal service, elegantly dressed in a green tail coat and top hat, and rewarded on his retirement in 1958 with the Royal Victorian Medal.

For the last sixteen years of his service, Bert Turp was Royal Gate Keeper at Wellington Arch. It had been moved to its present position by John Mowlem in 1884, the year before he was born, and there he lived, in bachelor comfort, on the north side, while the police occupied a small station on the south side.

'There is one occasion I remember very well. As you may know, only the reigning monarch is permitted to drive through the gates of Wellington Arch. When the King was coming back from Windsor, they used to tip me off – the journey took one hour – and I would open the gates for him. Well, this morning I got my usual message and opened up. At that moment, the late Duke of Kent, who was living in Belgrave Square, drove up in his sports car, and seeing the gates opened, nipped through just ahead of the King! There wasn't much I could do.

* The M.S.M. is no longer awarded for acts of gallantry in the field.

'That afternoon an equerry came up to see me and presented the King's apologies. He said that His Majesty was extremely annoyed and that "he had given His Royal Highness a good wigging".

'And then there was the Duke of Wellington across the way at Apsley House. As you know, I have this distinctive nose* and the police at Wellington Arch always called me "the Duke". Well, one day a valet comes over from Apsley House and says: "His Grace has heard about you and wants to meet you." "If he wants to borrow any money", I said, "I don't think I can oblige!" But no, – he wanted to see "the Duke", so I put on my uniform and polished my medals and presented myself the next afternoon. The Duke was delighted and we spent an hour together over a glass of beer. As I was going he said: "I've told my valet that if ever you feel like a drink, you're to come over here." I never have.'

In 1958, his eyesight failing, Bert Turp, gentleman Dragoon and farrier, retired. 'I should have applied to go into the Royal Hospital then, but I suppose I was stubborn and I sweated it out on my own in Pimlico.' But in 1965, nearly blind with a double cataract, he made the decision to go to Chelsea. He was in good hands; and within three years, his sight restored, he had taken a new lease of life.

R.S.M. Ives adds a humorous footnote: 'While he was waiting for his cataract operations, Bert Turp was cared for and led around by his friend, In-Pensioner Hughes. Came the day when he could put away his dark glasses, and we met outside the Orderly Room. He looked at me closely. "So *you're* the R.S.M.?" An even closer look. "I never knew you were so ugly!"'

At about the time In-Pensioner Turp enlisted in the Royals, a small boy, then aged two, was growing up in the back streets of Pendleton, near Salford, in Lancashire. George Batty was one of a family of four (his eldest brother Abraham was to become the much-respected head lad in Herbert Blagrave's stables). His father was a rolling stone, more often out of work than in, and young George was left to fend for himself. 'It was a hard life, but a happy one. We lived off bread and jam, or potatoes and gravy, and if I was good,

---

* In-Pensioner Turp, with his aquiline nose and pointed jaw, is a rare amalgam of the Iron Duke and Mr Punch.

my father used to give me the top of his egg as a special treat. I went to school at five and I suppose I must have done pretty well because for the last two years I was in X.7 which was as high as I could get.' His first job was driving a horse and cart for Threlfall's brewery – 'a real broken-down old thing with long whiskers and furry legs'. The job lasted one day and ended with a broken wrist. Next he donned a celluloid collar and went to work for a dye-company where, innocent of the fact that life is real and life is earnest, he was debagged by the female staff who oiled and greased what might be called his working parts. He began to grow up.

The outbreak of war in 1914 found him commuting on foot between Salford and Blackpool – it took him two days in each direction – there to carry parcels and sell papers and rock. Already he was determined to be a soldier. 'I used to see these men in hospital blue being driven about by ladies in posh cars and I was determined that I, too, would go out to the front and get wounded, though I was that simple, I really believed I would be able to dodge the shells and bullets!' It took him several months and all his persistence to be accepted and in the winter of 1915, still short of his sixteenth birthday, he became Pte Batty of the 23rd (Service) Battalion, Manchester Regiment. 'They gave us wooden rifles and a bit of drill, but no other training. I must have looked a proper baby and when we were at Felixstowe waiting to go over to France, I remember a man saying to me: "Do you change your own nappies?" I didn't care. I was a soldier now and that's all that mattered.

'In January, 1916 we sailed for Boulogne and spent a short time at Étaples where I fired my first rifle-course – fifteen rounds in all – and we were given some instruction in trench warfare.' Two weeks later Pte Batty was in the front line at Lavantie in the Festubert sector. He was lucky. He could well have found himself in a much hotter spot a few miles away at Loos.

He did not have to wait long for a taste of the real thing. With the opening of the Somme offensive on July 1, his division – the 35th – was transferred to the southern sector.

One summer we retraced by car his long, long trail – from Fleurbaix to Béthune (a bath and a clean shirt there in a brewery sadly lacking in beer), foot-slogging on to Albert and to Aveluy Wood, that dark and sinister place where troops assembled for 'the big push'. And so to Guillemont.

Liddell Hart has described it thus: 'Now a peaceful hamlet amid cornfields, it was then a shambles of blended horror and mystery. Except for Thiepval, no hamlet has exacted a heavier price for its possession.' Into this unspeakable place came the 23rd Manchesters. They were to lose three-quarters of their officers and men and it was to be an experience that George Batty will not easily forget. 'We seemed forever to be advancing and retiring across a hundred yards of mud and shell-holes, while the Germans in Trônes Wood fired at us in enfilade. Once I got my puttee caught on the wire and I remember being much more concerned about facing the Quartermaster with a torn puttee than being killed by German bullets. I remember, too, meeting a man in the sunken road whose arm was hanging by a shred and when he asked me to pull it off, I said I was sorry but I couldn't do that.' He was still barely sixteen.

Here, too, Pte Batty was platoon runner, carrying messages to the French at Combles, so he might fairly claim that for a while he was the right-hand man of the entire British Army on the Somme. Two miles to his left, at Mametz, In-Pensioner Rooney and In-Pensioner Mitchell were also heavily involved, while in front of Delville Wood, In-Pensioner Webb was gaining the rare Warrant Officer's distinction of a Military *Cross*, while a C.S.M. with the Royal Welsh Fusiliers. The Royal Hospital has its full quota of Somme veterans.

That summer's day we 'walked the course' together and reconstructed among the quiet cornfields the old front-line of fifty-eight years ago (in the cemetery at Guillemont Road Raymond Asquith lies buried) and we drove round to Longueval and Ginchy so that Pte Batty could get his first view of how he must have looked to the Germans all those years ago. He said very little. There was very little left to say.

From the Somme George Batty was transferred to Arras – 'I was still scruffy and dirty so I spent 5 francs on a bottle of *eau-de-cologne* to make me smell nice!' – and eventually wounded, he was evacuated to the base hospital where his age was discovered and he was sent home. The end of the war found him with the Army of Occupation near Cologne, politely sharing his rations with a cowed and hungry German family on whom he was billetted.

By 1919 he was a civilian again and looking for work. An encounter with a foreman at the margarine factory in Irlam went like this:

'Can you lay bricks?'
'No.'
'Can you lay eggs?'
'No, but I'll have a try!'

– and he was signed on, first digging holes in the ground and then working inside until, clouting a cheeky girl with a slab of margarine, he was fired.

He goes on. 'So I decided to join up again. I'd seen my Company Commander riding his horse while we trudged all the way to Albert and I made up my mind that I'd done enough walking. So I put in for the cavalry of the line. I was posted to the 9th Lancers in Tidworth and then sent on a draft to the 21st Lancers in India. I'd never been on a horse but the Army have a way of putting that right. They taught you the hard way and I can still remember my lance drill to this day. I can also remember being run away with by a brute of a horse, A.45, and nearly killed!'

In 1921 Trooper Batty, as he now was, came home. Ireland, a voyage to Chanak in Turkey ferrying cavalry horses, many of which died in transit, and then to the cavalry depôt at Canterbury where he met his future wife – 'I thought George sounded a bit common, so I told her my name was Gerald, and Gerry I became!'

The Battys' service life proceeded along a conventional pattern: Egypt, a second tour in India (now with two small camp-followers), transfer to the 3rd Hussars in Tidworth at the time of mechanization, and so to civvy street in 1938.

'When the war came I eventually got a job as a valet at the Savoy, £3 a week plus tips and learning the ropes by trial and error. There's the old joke about "what the butler saw". That goes for a valet, too! You meet all sorts – and you get some surprises. I remember Nasser, who was unknown then, getting me to line up the floor staff and handing us each a fiver. There was the day I nearly got shot by General Dolittle's bodyguard. And there were occasions over which I had better draw a veil.'

After eight years at the Savoy, he moved to the Hyde Park Hotel where his charges included Winston Churchill, Lord Ismay, Elizabeth Taylor and Michael Wilding, and the Sultan of Zanzibar. Good soldier that he is, his lips are sealed!

Finally, he went for his last three working years to the Cavalry Club, a round peg unusually accommodated at the end in a round hole. When, in 1970, his wife died, he came to Chelsea. 'It was the saving of me. I don't know what I would have done otherwise. And I think that's true of many other men in the Hospital. You want for nothing here and some of the old stagers have no idea how life has changed outside. Do you remember that old song from the first war – "I'm alright in my little dug-out"? Well, that goes for me now.'

They are two of many – old gentlemen with long memories, natural courtesy, and a cheerful disposition which has survived some rugged experiences. If they may be thought lucky, it is only because 'by their good deservings' they have earned the right to be sheltered from the harsh winds that blow outside. *In subsidium et levamen emeritorum senio belloque fractorum* . . .

14
Soldiering on

❦

It is a place for all seasons; genial under the summer sun, the lighted Wards welcoming and warm in a winter's dusk. As it has survived its troubled past, so it has mellowed and grown old with the same dignity which age has lent to its veteran soldiers, for there is a quality about the Royal Hospital not shared by any other of our traditional institutions.

It is no place for the unromantic. The old gentlemen, whether in homely blue or formal scarlet, are a present and constant link with the past, and the veterans of Mons and Alamein worship in the same chapel, sit at the same dining-tables, and take their ease in the same Colonnade as the ghosts of Ramillies and Fontenoy, of Plassey, Albuera and Inkerman. The battle honours inscribed on the panels of the Great Hall tell the enduring story of the British Army; but the old soldiers are themselves the living embodiment of that story. This sense of continuity informs and underlies the special quality of Chelsea.

The evidence of the In-Pensioners before the Belper Committee of 1894 quoted in an earlier chapter is a case in point. It would not be difficult to take each of those men – humorous, forthright, melancholy, withdrawn, or plain spiky – and match him exactly to a Chelsea Pensioner of 1974. Old 'Peeping Tom' Barlow from Coventry has his living counterpart in ... but that would be betraying a confidence! Men do not change, least of all old men. Soldiers of a century ago laughed at the same bawdy jokes and created the same mountains of complaint out of the same molehills of irritation. It is the world around them that has changed and who shall say whether for better or worse? Now at least In-Pensioner Wilson would not have to negotiate 1,080 stairs a day in order to smoke his pipe; but we may rest assured that he would find some equally vexatious aspect of Hospital life.

Yet if we dig a little deeper we can find some subtle differences. Between the old and the merely elderly at Chelsea today there is a distinction, difficult to define but nonetheless real. It has been suggested – not too fancifully either – that it is the difference between men who soldiered with horses and those who served in a mechanized army. This implies no criticism of the later vintage but simply illustrates how men absorb and reflect the temper of the time in which they have lived. Talking with In-Pensioners it is often difficult to remember that some of them have spent upwards of thirty years in civilian occupations since leaving the army, and yet they step back into new uniforms and old attitudes as if the intervening years had never been. As one of them neatly put it: 'When you pull out the plug, you never see where the bathwater goes.'

The Royal Hospital is unusual in another sense. It is neither a barrack nor an old people's home. The In-Pensioners are neither serving soldiers nor retired civilians. Their scarlet coats at once confer privileges and impose obligations on them, for these coats are a singular badge of honour and not simply a picturesque survival from another age. When Matthew Ingram obtained King James's permission that his pensioners should wear the royal livery, he may well have had in mind the military associations of the old religious orders. This might surprise the In-Pensioners of today but it comes close to explaining the nature of their institution.

Why then is there no long waiting-list for admission to the Royal Hospital? This is nothing new. A hundred years ago the annual average of applications was never more than 200, a tiny fraction of those qualified for entry. The figure is no greater today.

There are several possible reasons. The first is a question of human nature. Old people are notoriously, often stubbornly, independent, determined to end their days in old remembered places and surrounded by such personal treasures as they possess. It is partly a matter of pride, partly of fear, for the old have long memories and the poor-house still casts its long, dark shadow. But sometimes it is small, seemingly irrelevant things that tip the scale. James Taylor, aged 83, late 9th Lancers, who nursed an ailing wife at his North London home until the day she died, is a typical example. The conversation went like this:

'Are you happy living here? – Not since Hilda died.
'Are you comfortable? – I've known worse.
'Any money problems? – No, no money problems.
'Any family to go to? – No.
'Any friends? – No, not really. All the old ones are dead.
'How do you spend your time? – Reading, watching telly, mucking about in general. I don't drink, so I don't go to the pubs.

'Have you ever been to the Royal Hospital? – Oh yes, I used to go there quite a bit. It's a nice place and I had two chums there, but they're both gone.

'Why don't you apply to go there? You'd enjoy it.

'*A long pause. Then* – I've thought about it – *another pause* – but what would I do with my dog?'

Four months later James Taylor was dead.

A second reason is the Welfare State. A hundred years ago some In-Pensioners were prepared to face the rigours of life outside for the prospect of as little as 2*s.* a day and even the militant Mr Punter was campaigning for an additional 'age pension' at the turn of the century. But today, as we have seen, not many old soldiers come to Chelsea because the shoe is pinching too hard. The compulsions are different and the decisions more personal.

Yet the greatest single reason why Out-Pensioners stay outside is a widespread ignorance and prejudice about the nature and purpose of the Royal Hospital. The critics are invariably uninformed, the gossips usually malicious; but the reputation of the bad old days has lingered on. To many old men the image of the Hospital is still that of the poor-house and the In-Pensioners objects to be pitied rather than envied. To others, it is a military institution whose inmates are subjected to strict discipline precisely because they *are* old soldiers. And to these and hundreds like them, admission to Chelsea is tantamount to an act of surrender.

These prejudices are without any kind of foundation either in fact – or fancy. If the Royal Hospital is a glorified poor-house, then the quicker we build a few more like it the better. If the In-Pensioners are ruled with a rod of iron, then it is the most flexible piece of disciplinary metal yet devised. And if admission to the Royal Hospital means the surrender of personal liberty, consider the tale of In-Pensioner Paltridge, late 17/21st Lancers, who, having won £1,500 on the football pools, galloped off on a three-months' world cruise.

It has been called 'the finest hotel in the world'. It is a very fair description. But more exactly it is one of the stateliest *homes* of England. Here, in their village setting, the old soldiers enjoy the privacy to which they are entitled, but they keep open house and visitors – especially the ladies – will find that the age of chivalry is by no means dead. And those who penetrate as far as the In-Pensioners' Club will discover that it is not only charity that begins at home.

The village has its problems and its imperfections like any other community. Familiarity often breeds contempt and old age can sometimes be very crabbed indeed, while at the other end of the scale the voice of authority is sometimes unimaginative and tactless. Let a wise old gentleman, with the black humour of his kind, have the last word: 'I can't think of a grander place to come and die.' Or, he might have added, to find a new lease of life.

The future is unpredictable. It has never been otherwise at the Royal Hospital. But we can indulge in a little crystal-gazing.

In the short term, life in the village will continue with little outward and visible change, the old gentlemen secure in the knowledge that they are sustained by the respect and affection of the public at large. But time bears all its sons away. The first to go will be the last of the old South Africa men, and after them the dwindling company of Old Contemptibles. What then if the gaps in the ranks are not filled? What if the numbers decline and the Long Wards lie empty?*

It has been argued that admission to the Hospital should presently be extended to pensioners of the Royal Navy and the Royal Air Force. To do so would be a mistake, for it might well create more problems than it solved. And what of women pensioners? When Charles referred in his Royal Warrant to 'land souldiers' it could not have occurred to him that the day of the Amazons would come – much, we may be sure, to the merry monarch's delight. It is a fascinating prospect on which it would be impolitic to speculate too closely.

How safe is the Royal Hospital from outside predators? In 1875 the entire property was conveyed by Act of Parliament to the Chelsea Commissioners in trust for ever; but what one Act can join together, another can put asunder. Envious eyes have already been cast at Wren's 'stately fabrick' as the natural setting for some soulless educational establishment or even a dormitory for bureaucrats, and the open spaces of Ranelagh Gardens and the South Grounds offer tempting possibilities for the apostles of the high-rise society. The In-Pensioners would be well-advised to keep their

* At April 1, 1974. The number of In-Pensioners was 398.

bayonets sharpened and their powder dry. They may one day be called upon to man their barricades.

When, on January 30, 1708, the Earl of Orford petitioned for the recovery of the lease of his 'Dwelling and Garden' at the Royal Hospital, the Chelsea Commissioners replied to him thus:

> 'Wee dare not advise the granting away by Lease or otherwise any part of the Lands of the said Hospital which, haveing been given by the Royall Founder to a use so pious in its selfe, so advantageous as well as honourable to the publick, Wee hope will always be preserv'd Sacred and Intire.'

Amen to that.

Index

A Village in Chelsea

Somerset Light Infantry, 78
South Sea Bubble, 136; Company,
    123, 128
Staker, I/P Charles, 170
standing orders, first, 114
Suffolk Regt., 78
Sutcliffe, Matthew, Dean of Exeter,
    60

Taylor, James, 214–15
Templer, Field Marshal Sir Gerald,
    195–6
Tessier, Dr, 145
Test Acts, 30, 78
Thom, I/P John, 170
tobacco ration, 204
Townsend, Capt. Bill, 179
Turp, I/P Bertram, 14, 175, 205–8
Tuston, Thomas, later Earl of
    Thanet, 73

Upnor Castle, 102

Vanbrugh, Sir John, 81, 137
Venner, 43
Vivian, Hon. J. C., M.P., 167
voluntary co-operation, as under-
    lying philosophy at Chelsea
    Royal Hospital, 201

Walpole, Horace, 139, 143
Walpole, Robert, 18–19, 21, 119,
    121, 131, 132, 134, 135–8, 143,
    147
West Yorkshire Regt., 78
Whalley, Edward, 41
Whelan, I/P John, 170

Whitwood, Ciprian, 109
Wilford, General R. R., 21, 160,
    164
William III, King, 36, 38, 73 n., 88,
    94, 97–8, 101, 102, 118
Wilson, I/P Hugh, 170, 176, 213
Windham, William, 106, 131, 134,
    156
Windham Act (1806), 156–7
Winks, Thomas, 109
Wise, Henry, 103
Worcester, battle of, 41
Wray, Sir Cecil, 154
Wren, Sir Christopher, designs
    Royal Hospital, 17, 21, 66–8,
    70–2, 76, 80–1, 83, 98, 100–1;
    designs Farley alms-house and
    Church, 45; proposes demolition
    of Chelsea College, 60; vote of
    thanks to, 61; birth and career,
    63, 65; designer of St Paul's
    Cathedral, 65, 119, 124;
    appointed as architect of Royal
    Hospital, 65; has doubts on
    accession of James II, 76;
    proposes revenue for Hospital,
    79; designs house and garden for
    Ranelagh, 89, 90; takes final
    steps to bring Hospital into use,
    103–4; draws up Instruction
    Book, 109; seeks to avoid con-
    frontation with Ranelagh, 116;
    builds Royal Naval Hospital,
    118, 124; his affection for
    Chelsea, 118; requests additional
    money for pensioners, 128
Wyatt, William, 47